HOW TO TRAIN LIKE YOUR LIF[

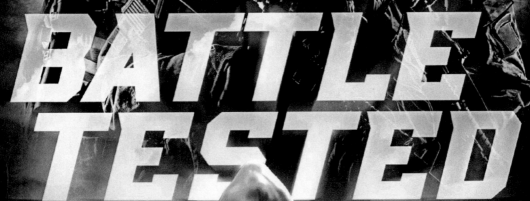

BATTLE TESTED

ARLO GAGESTEIN
CSCS, LMT

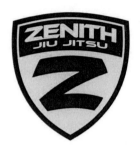
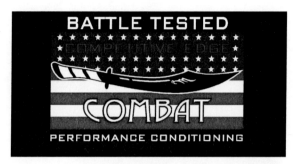
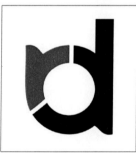

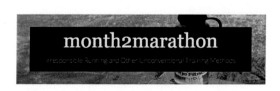

Table of Contents

One Warrior's Creed

If today is to be THE DAY, so be it.

If you seek to do battle with me this day you will receive the best that I am capable of giving.

It may not be enough, but it will be everything that I have to give and it will be impressive for I have constantly prepared myself for this day.

I have trained, drilled and rehearsed my actions so that I might have the best chance of defeating you.

I have kept myself in peak physical condition, schooled myself in the martial skills and have become proficient in the application of combat tactics.

You may defeat me, but you will pay a severe price and will be lucky to escape with your life.

You may kill me, but I am willing to die if necessary.

I do not fear Death, for I have been close enough to it on enough occasions that it no longer concerns me.

But I do fear the loss of my Honor and would rather die fighting than to have it said that I was without Courage.

So I WILL FIGHT YOU, no matter how insurmountable it may seem, and to the death if need be, in order that it may never be said of me that I was not a Warrior.

Steven R. Watt, All Rights Reserved

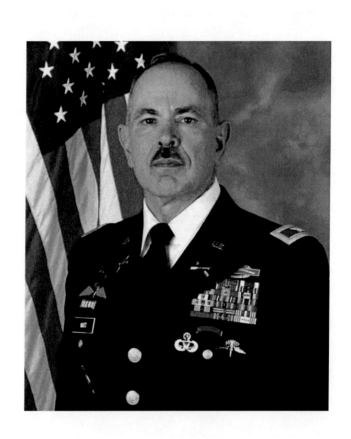

Foreword - Colonel (Ret.) Steven R. Watt

As a martial artist, street police officer, SWAT Team member, and Special Forces soldier, I have long understood the relationship between physical fitness and surviving a fight. Whether armed or unarmed, one's ability to survive the initial attack, respond appropriately and effectively enough to come out alive, and then recover from the post-combat effects, is predicated on one's level of physical fitness. What I didn't really understand, until multiple tours in Afghanistan and Iraq, was the connection between physical and mental fitness. One's ability to survive long-term, well past combat and combat conditions, is founded on mental resilience.

You'll notice I don't refer to "winning" a fight. In the real world, off the mats and outside of competition where there are no rules and surviving means living through the ordeal, it's not over when the enemy flees, capitulates, or dies. It's over when your mind has come to peace with the event. For some it can be fairly immediate while for others it may take extended time. Some are never over it and are so impacted by it they ultimately self-destruct.

The key, learned in combat as a Special Forces soldier and as a SWAT officer, is that individuals with high levels of physical fitness are far more mentally prepared not only for the fight but for the aftermath. As a general rule, the greater one's level of physical fitness the greater one's ability to handle stress of all kinds. Physical stress, mental stress, emotional stress, those are the realms of the Warrior. Highly physically fit people perform better under all kinds of stress, including being under fire, than those who aren't. Highly physically fit people tend to have the greater mental resiliency necessary for defeating the hidden enemy inside one's mind and surviving the aftermath of extreme life-threatening events. Hence the demand by all high-performance combat units that members be very physically fit.

I met Arlo through police officers friends who were attending his fitness courses at Competitive Edge Fitness in Ogden, Utah. Arlo gave me a copy of his first book, Warrior Core: Core Training Secrets for the Modern Combat Athlete, which I read immediately. I had studied fitness at the FBI National Academy, the Cooper Institute, through the 3rd SFG(A)'s THOR III program, and during intense personal studies. I had attended numerous specialized fitness training events and had developed a fitness philosophy geared toward Warriorhood, what I felt was necessary in terms of a formula for training to produce physical and mental Warrior attributes. It became clear in a very short period of time that Arlo knows how to build highly fit and resilient Warriors.

I strongly recommend Arlo's latest book, Battle Tested. In it you'll find not only techniques for high-level physical and mental Warrior training, but also the foundational knowledge required for understanding the means of obtaining training success. Arlo will give you the "why" and the "how" in language easily understood. Of course, you'll have to take it from there and apply it for yourself. Only you can determine how far you go, at what speed, and to what end. Arlo can, and will, provide the means, you'll have to provide the commitment.

Coming out of a tour of Iraq in the summer of 2007, I was reflecting on the many SWAT Officers and Special Operators I had known through both of my careers and was wondering how I would explain "us" to those who had little idea of what we had gone through to get to where we were, what we were willing to do, and why we dedicate ourselves to a life of continual training. I wrote something I titled One Warrior's Creed and it is contained in this book. As you'll notice, keeping oneself in "peak physical condition" is a requirement for Warriors in order to be prepared for "The Day." Arlo, and this book, can be a part of your initial, or continuing, journey on the path to Warriorhood. I hope to see you along the way.

Steven R. Watt (Randy)
Colonel (Ret.), U.S. Army Special Forces
Chief of Police
Ogden, Utah, Police Department

PART I
The Making of a Warrior

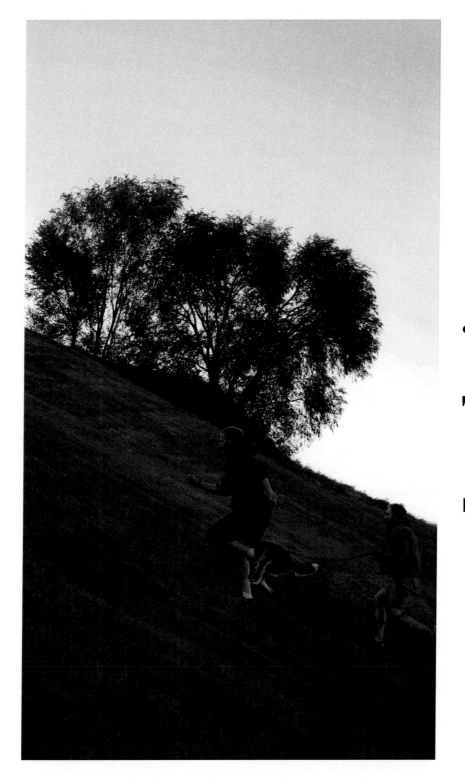

Introduction
Are You Ready?

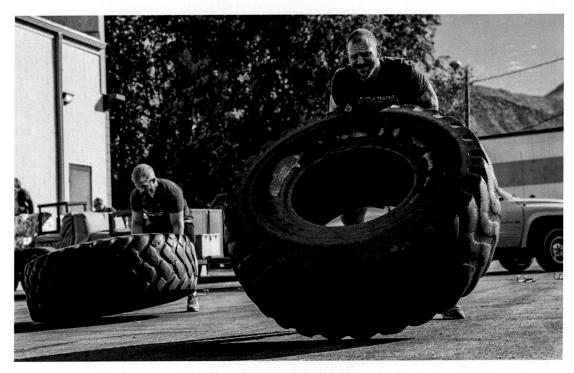

Introduction – Are You Ready?

"Where there's discomfort, there's fear, in these very tough positions, you're in a little piece of hell. And through this daily suffering, you learn to survive in these situations. You have to find comfort in uncomfortable situations. You have to be able to live in your worst nightmare. Jiu-jitsu puts you completely in the moment where you must have complete focus on finding a solution to the problem. This trains the mind to build that focus, to increase your awareness, your capacity to solve problems. Sometimes, you don't have to win. You cannot win. But that has nothing to do with losing."
- Rickson Gracie

Get comfortable being uncomfortable!

People get very caught up in comfort and in routine. Even people who will intentionally work themselves to a point of stumbling out of the gym are susceptible to it. They believe they are killing themselves in the gym, yet it is very well premeditated to keep them in their comfort zone. I see people stuck on body part splits, who religiously work their chest on Monday year after year. These same people won't lift anything they did yesterday because they are sore and it doesn't fit their training schedule. There are people everywhere who have convinced themselves they can't get a good workout in if they forgot to bring their pre-workout blend.

Before we begin, you should understand that my goal in writing this book is not to make your life easy and predictable. My entire objective is to shake your routine up and get you training outside of your comfort zone. I anticipate and hope that there will be times you curse me and wonder what inspired you to give *Battle Tested* a shot. Some days will be fun, some challenging, some downright miserable.

So why are you reading this? How did I convince you to abandon your favorite routine for something likely to be extremely difficult that may occasionally leave you nauseous? Because deep down, you know that you can be better. You know that you can challenge yourself a little bit more, that you are capable of a little more than you thought, that by leaving your comfort zone you will grow physically, mentally, and perhaps spiritually.

Also you love to be challenged. You relish the thought of working harder than anyone else is working. You thrive on the knowledge that few people are capable of the things you do, and that most would be terrified by the thought of even trying. How do I know this? I am like you. We are drawn to people similar to ourselves and to ideas similar to our own. We are drawn to those who are never satisfied with their current abilities. Those who want to push the envelope, to dance on the edge of possible and crazy.

In his book *Band of Brothers* about legendary Easy Company, 506th Regiment, 101st Airborne in WWII, Steven E. Ambrose explains that these people volunteered to jump out of airplanes for two profound, personal reasons,

> ''The desire to be better than the other guy took hold. Each man in his own way had gone through what Richard Winters experienced; a realization that doing his best was a better way of getting through the Army than hanging around with the sad excuses for soldiers they met in the recruiting depots or basic training. They wanted to make their Army time positive, a learning and maturing and challenging experience. Second, they knew they were going into combat, and they did not want to go in with poorly trained, poorly conditioned, poorly motivated draftees on either sided of them. As to choosing between being a paratrooper spearheading the offensive and an ordinary infantryman who could not trust the guy next to him, they decided the greater risk was with the infantry. When the shooting started, they wanted to look up to the guy beside them, not down.''

Those who join the *Battle Tested* tribe will do so because they have heart. They have the will and the drive that will inspire the rest of us to be better, to work harder, to strive for greatness. They know working harder than anyone else will serve them better now and in the long run. It will protect them in moments of combat and better prepare them to meet any challenge in life. We want to go into battle with like-minded, well-prepared, well-conditioned warriors at our side. Warriors we can trust with our lives if need be.

Ambrose goes on to say, "Not that they knew much about airborne, except that it was new and all-volunteer. They had been told that the physical training was tougher than anything they had ever seen, or that any other unit in the Army would undergo, but these young lions were eager for that. They expected that, when they were finished with their training they would be bigger, stronger, tougher than when they started, and would have gone through the training with the guys who would be fighting beside them."

As combat athletes, we want to train with people who will bring out the best in us. If we are always the fastest, strongest, scariest, or most talented athlete in the gym, there is little motivation to improve. It may be good for your ego, but you are selling yourself short. However,when we are challenged and pushed by others with a similar mindset and willingness to suffer to become better, it is necessary for us to work harder to keep from falling behind. Mark Twight, founder of Gym Jones puts it best on his website where he explains why his gym is invitation only:

'We invite athletes of a certain temperament and ability to train here because they foster the environment we prefer. It is difficult to improve while training exclusively with less capable practitioners. Talented athletes surround themselves with others of a similar or higher caliber - both mental and physical - and improve by doing so.'

If you are ready - ready to put yourself to the test, ready to train harder and to be better than the opposition, ready to suffer for the greater good - then please, read on and prepare to get comfortable being uncomfortable!

Below, you will find your first *Immediate Action Step*. Throughout this book you will find these action steps. They are quick, easy tasks that will propel you forward on your journey toward greatness. Taking action is an essential step toward success, so when you come to these in the book, don't think, "Oh, I will come back to this later." No. Wherever you are, follow the instructions immediately and take action now. You will already be one step ahead of most people by taking immediate action.

IMMEDIATE ACTION #1

Are You Up For The Challenge?

If you fit the mold, and are ready to suffer with us for the greater good, **join the Battle Tested Tribe.**

Battle Tested Tribe is a secret group on Facebook for those who have purchased Battle Tested. You should have received an invitation to the group within 1-2 days of ordering the book. If you did not, please e-mail battletestedbook@gmail.com

We are here to build community and help each other along the journey toward greatness. We will be posting videos, photos, training tips, etc. We also encourage dialogue, progress posts, and questions from you, the readers. We are excited to have you - welcome to our tribe!

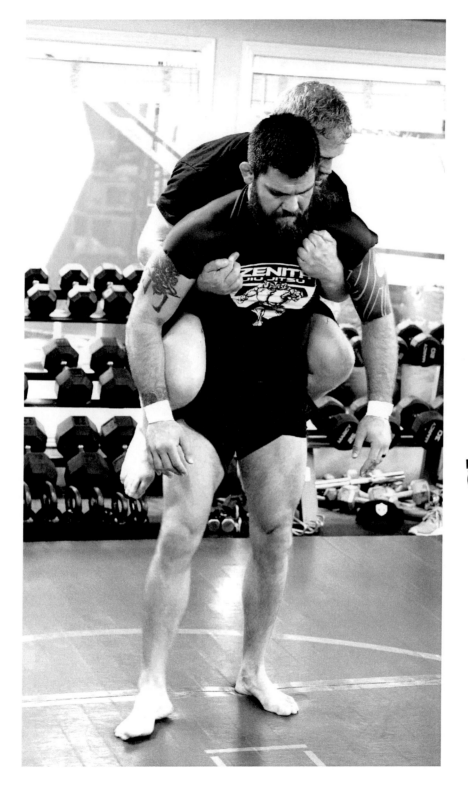

Chapter 1
Preparation is Key

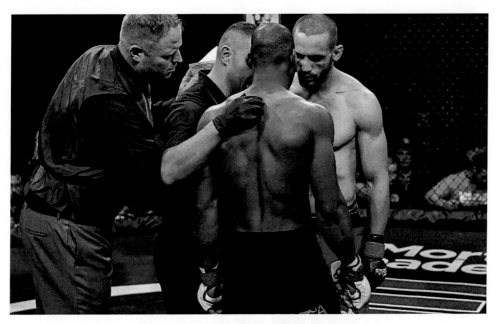

Chapter 1 - Preparation is Key

war·ri·or (wôr′ē-ər) *n.*
1. *One who is engaged in or experienced in battle.*
2. *One who is engaged aggressively or energetically in an activity, cause, or conflict.*

This book is written for warriors. While true that our primary audience are soldiers and fighters, many athletes' well-being and even lives depend on their preparation. The soldier, the police officer, the firefighter, the MMA fighter, the climber, all benefit greatly from training like their life depends on it. And in many cases, it does. This book is written for elite military operators. This book is written for the grunts. This book is written for professional MMA fighters. This book is written for the guy who just wants to step in the cage once. This book is written for the experienced mountaineer with sights set on Everest. This book is written for the recreational athlete determined to run their first half marathon.

Aren't their careers completely different? Don't fighters have time to prepare for a predetermined opponent, on a predetermined date, at a predetermined time, while soldiers need to be ready at all times, not knowing with whom or when they may be fighting to the death? Don't mountaineers know in plenty of time when they will arrive at base camp?

The answer is of course, yes, but when the event arrives, the outcome is plagued with uncertainty.

We hope for the best, but prepare for the worst, because that is necessary. As Archilochus said, "We do not rise to the level of our expectations. We fall to the level of our training." We choose to train our fighters like our soldiers, our climbers like our grapplers, so that they too are prepared for anything at any time. If our Battle Tested fighters are ever out of shape and need several months of intense physical preparation for an upcoming fight, we did something wrong. Sure depending on the opponent and his/her strengths, you should tweak your strength and conditioning plan, and of course you'll taper the workload leading up to a fight, but our goal is that as a Battle Tested athlete, you will always be ready and prepared to adapt to the unexpected.

So why train soldiers and fighters together? It is really about heart and physical preparedness. We choose to train warriors. We don't choose to separate them into different classifications. Sure we adjust training variables based on their job, but we train all our athletes to be warriors. True warriors know their success is in the mind. The physical training variables can easily be manipulated and adjusted, the real training happens in the mind. These warriors need to be physically and mentally prepared for battle at all times. If our warriors are able to persevere when the going gets tough, to press on when the outcome looks sketchy at best, to keep coming at the opponent regardless of the circumstances, regardless of how fatigued they might be, if they are better mentally prepared – these warriors will do well either on the battlefield or in the cage.

The Survival Readiness Triangle

A colleague, Randy Watt, of Warrior Creed (www.warriorcreed.us), introduced me to the Survival Readiness Triangle. Randy is Ogden City police chief, former SWAT commander, and former commander of the 19th Special Forces Group. The idea is that there

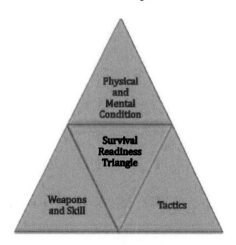

are three important components to being able to survive a life or death situation.

The top portion of the triangle is Physical and Mental Condition. The bottom left corner is Weapons/Skill and the bottom right is Tactics. The top portion of the triangle is Physical and Mental Condition. If you are lacking in one of these areas, you are 33% less likely to survive a hostile situation. If you are lacking in two areas, you are 66% less likely to survive.

That being said, the pinnacle of the triangle is physical and mental condition. Battle Tested is written to address this portion of your survival readiness. If you are a fighter, you already have a coach responsible for skill and tactics, a soldier and you learn these things in the military. You also likely have reasonable physical and mental condition. We still intend to improve it.

Regardless of your profession, you need to train to survive. In his book 100 Deadly Skills: Survival Edition, retired SEAL, Clint Emerson, says, "If you don't have the physical conditioning necessary to get yourself out of trouble, the skills in this book won't do you much good." He continues, "Whether you're exiting a burning building or knocking an assailant unconscious, the ordeal will consist of surmounting the initial crisis and then running or crawling your way to safe ground some distance away."

When your life depends on it, will YOU be ready?

In The Arena
Finding Order In Chaos

On a cold, snow covered January day, Narcotics Agents were serving a residential, knock and announce search warrant. With no response from within, agents proceeded to enter the house. As they did, their world erupted into chaos, as a suspect waiting inside the home opened fire.

Prior to this day, one of the agents, Agent T, had 12 years of law enforcement experience, including five years of SWAT training and experience. He had 100's of hours of firearms and tactical police training and had been in numerous high-stress tactical situations where shots were fired. His fitness was on point as he'd been working out diligently for 15 years and had also trained Jiu-Jitsu obsessively for the past three years.

Now, in an instant, he and 10 other officers were in the middle of an unexpected ambush that ultimately left one officer dead and five others with gunshot wounds. During the next 19 minutes, many things happened, much of which Agent T does not remember. When the firing started, he exited the house with several members of the team, following one officer out who had been shot in the face. Not seeing all the officers, Agent T went back toward the door to find the other agents involved. Bullets started flying again and Agent T quickly took cover behind a car, then circled around the front of the house and took cover by some bushes beyond a small hill where he could see the front door. He realized he was in a tactically horrible position because there was a patrol car in the road with the lights directly on him, exposing him to being seen by the suspect inside of the home.

This is where the details get blurred. Agent T believed he then ran in front of the house, past the car and up to another house to the south where he could see the door that they initially entered. He remembers being there with his gun at the ready pointing toward the door for about 5 minutes. At some point he believed he was being shot at again and ran to turn off the car lights because he saw other officers in front of the car. Agent T believed he ran back to the car and opened the door to shut off the lights.

Video evidence and accounts of other involved officers later showed that this wasn't the case. Agent T has no recollection of lying in the roadway behind the curb attempting to cover two injured officers on the ground. The 5 minutes he thought he spent covering the door from the house to the south, on video, ended up being less then 10 seconds before he is moving again. He also doesn't recall grabbing another injured officer's extra key en route to opening the patrol car to turn off the lights. Once he has the key and is running back to the car he and the other officers ARE shot at again and Agent T jumps on the road behind the car. While he doesn't remember this, it explains the scratch marks he later finds on the side of his gun.

Research has shown that incomplete or fragmented details of traumatic events are very common. Simultaneously, people involved in traumatic events often recall other details with extraordinary accuracy. Agent T remembers a conversation with another officer who

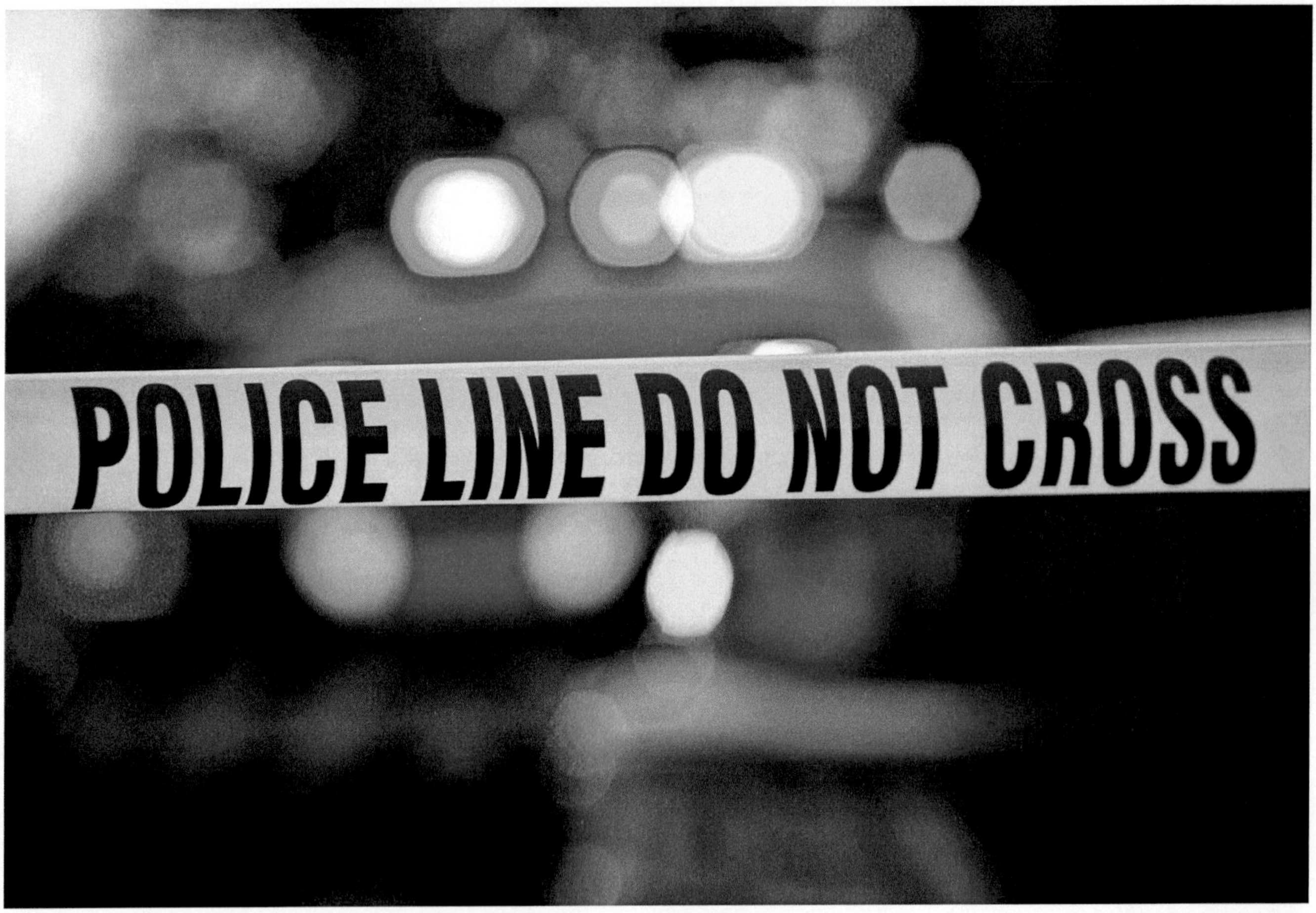
POLICE LINE DO NOT CROSS

collapsed next to him behind the patrol car clear as day. "Are you hit? Where?"

After turning off the lights, Agent T ran across the yard to drag another officer an estimated 40 yards to the roadway and instinctively placed the officer behind the engine block of the patrol car for protection. Agent T then started loading other injured officers in the car. Ambulances will not come to the scene during an active shooting, so all injured officers had to be evacuated in police vehicles. Of the 11 officers, 6 were shot. Tragically, one agent did not survive.

Of the details Agent T remembers, one thing is clear, "What I vividly recall though, is complete and utter exhaustion. This was a 19-minute gun battle that seemed to have lasted hours in my head. My legs were quivering and my back was aching. I had that adrenaline dump that you could just never imagine. To put it in the right mindset is to see one of your friends or family members murdered, and all of these people who you care for deeply, looking like they are going to die."

"This is what I think about: I would say at the time, that I was in superior physical shape and had a higher caliber training than the vast majority of officers employed at my police department. And I was smoked. Absolutely, completely, physically and mentally drained. What if I wasn't in that great of shape? What if I wasn't that prepared? What could have gone worse than that already, bottom line, zero, absolute worst experience. Well it could have been worse. We had 6 officers shot and only one died. So I don't know. I think about dragging one of the officers back. Would I have made it? Could I have made it? I don't know. But I did. There is a lot to learn from it."

In reality, during the chaos, Agent T performed his job better than he perceived. The things he actually did, but does not recall, he truly believes it is due to his training and experience. "I credit my police training, tactical training, Jiu-Jitsu training, and my gym time to making some correct decisions when even to this day it is a complete blank. So basically, when I'm on autopilot, I'm doing the right things in those situations. And I credit that 100% to the preparation prior. That is why I'm a huge proponent of A, training, training correctly, and B, physically training. When I'm telling other law enforcement officers the importance of training and fitness, I wish that they could understand. Unfortunately, for me to understand the outcome, I had to go through it. Everything went wrong. Literally everything. And there were some heroic acts on a lot of people's parts that night. I am surrounded by my real-life heroes. Not a lot of people can say that. But we have to learn from our mistakes. We have to get better. And we have to NEVER let that happen again. Ever."

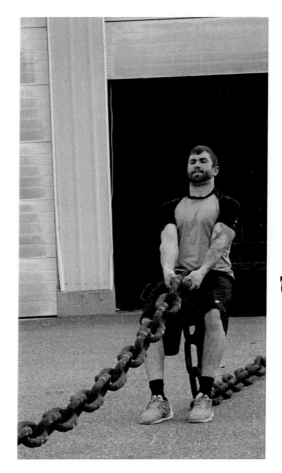

Chapter 2
Training the Body

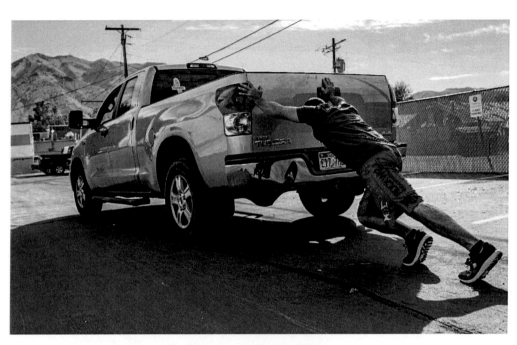

Chapter 2 – Training the Body

"The goal of physical training can be summed up in one phrase, "to make yourself as indestructible as possible." The harder a man is to kill, the longer he will remain effective, as a climber, a soldier, or what ever."
-Mark Twight

A 1993 study at the University of Miami, Ohio found physical fitness to be the number one predictor of shooting accuracy. That alone is a reason to make physical training a priority if you are a soldier or police officer. Your body needs to be a stable platform for your firearm to place the rounds where you want them. At a tactical strength and conditioning conference I went to, Frank Palkoska, the Division Chief of the U.S. Army Physical Readiness Division prioritized the physical training components for a soldier as the overlap of mobility, strength, and endurance. Speed, agility, and power are additional aspects of fitness that benefit both the soldier and the fighter. It is important to realize however that speed, agility, and power require a good base of flexibility, stability, and strength as renowned physiotherapist Paul Chek points out. He places components of fitness and performance on a continuum, noting that certain attributes of physical fitness need to be present before developing others.

Flexibility - Stability - Strength - Power - Speed

Obviously the fighter needs exceptional fitness as well. Because the needs of the soldier and the grappler or MMA fighter are so varied, we felt it important to stray from traditional training, and focus on strategies that include it all. Certainly a fighter benefits from being stronger than his opponent. Likewise being faster, or more explosive gives the athlete an advantage. But, a fighter also needs the muscular endurance to go all-out non-stop for three to five 5-minute rounds as well without losing strength, focus, or motivation due to fatigue.

The same is true of the soldier who may have to travel non-stop days on end through the jungle or desert, only to become engaged in close-quarter combat when being able to quickly and violently overcome an opponent is a matter of life and death. Endurance is essential, strength is essential, power is essential, balance is essential, speed and agility are essential.

Training strength and endurance together is known as concurrent training, and is thought less than ideal by some people in the strength and conditioning industry. While some studies suggest traditional periodization is better than concurrent training, other research indicates the opposite is true and would counter that concurrent training is ideal for military populations. Would I train a high jumper concurrently? Probably not. I am a firm believer that the training should mimic the demands of the job. We need to evaluate the job or event, assess individual strengths and weaknesses, and design a practical program from there.

Evaluating the demands on a soldier make it obvious that concurrent training is ideal. It is ideal for competitive fighters as well. I have been training my athletes concurrently for more than 10 years with extraordinary results. Can we make athletes stronger by taking them through a dedicated strength mesocycle? Perhaps. But this would likely come at the cost of a decrease in necessary endurance. Conversely, focusing 100% on endurance will also result in a decrease in strength. Without a predictable dedicated in-season, concurrent training is realistic and practical. A warrior needs to be ready at all times.

Durability

Durability is our number one priority while training a warrior. An injured MMA fighter does not fight. An injured soldier is a liability to the team. An injured police officer is put on light duty. A fighter of any kind must be very resilient if they intend to have a long career. Several things play into physical durability or resilience to the outward demands that a warrior's career demands of their body. As Palkoska stated, mobility, stability, strength, and endurance are priorities and all are important components of durability. Lacking in any of these areas will make an athlete more at risk for injury as well as decrease their ability to perform at a high level for a sustained period of time.

Mobility/Stability

When a joint lacks either mobility or stability, there is a greater risk of injury. Interestingly, the joint that is lacking said mobility or stability is often not where the pain shows up. An athlete with poor hip mobility for example might be dealing with knee pain.

This makes it important to consider the cause of pain whenever having symptoms. Ice and rest may help a sore knee, but if the root cause is your hip, it will continue to be an issue until the hip mobility is addressed. As Ida Rolf, founder of Rolfing explains, "Joints become the red flags; they tell you if and how something is wrong. You have to look for relationship, not only of the joints, but within all of the mesodermal tissue."

As a general guideline from the ground up, joint segments alternate the need for mobility and stability, and pain at one joint might originate at that joint as in the case of an injury (meniscus damage, ligament strain, etc.) or may originate from the level above or below the pain sight. This of course varies on an individual basis, which we will cover later in this book. For the vast majority of people, this chart would be a good place to start.

JOINT LEVEL	TRAINING GOAL
Ankle	Increase Mobility
Knee	Increase Stability
Hip	Increase Mobility
Lumbar Spine	Increase Stability
Thoracic Spine	Increase Mobility
Shoulder (Glenohumeral)	Increase Stability
Shoulder (Scapulothoracic)	Increase Mobility
Shoulder (Acromioclavicular)	Increase Stability
Cervical Spine	Increase Mobility

A joint without sufficient mobility limits natural movement both at the joint and changes the movement pattern at the surrounding joints. A joint without sufficient stability is more susceptible to injury and also creates what world-renowned physical therapist, Gray Cook, refers to as energy leaks, allowing potential power to dissipate from the joint, limiting its strength and function.

Strength

It is no secret that strength improves performance. I also believe that many injuries are a result of the athlete not being strong enough. With limited strength, the athlete lacks the joint stability required for load bearing work. Great strength, however, can protect susceptible sites against injury. After surgery for a shattered tibial plateau, my brother, Arlan, literally went several years unknowingly without an ACL (anterior cruciate ligament). He was backcountry skiing, racing mountain bikes and lifting hard in the gym, all with nagging knee pain, but still functioning at a high level. Eventually he went back under the knife to clean out his knee and they realized he had no trace of an ACL left. A torn, or in this case, non-existent ACL leaves a knee incredibly unstable, but my brother's legs were so strong that they

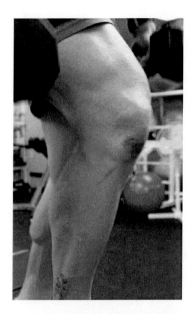

Years of cycling and skiing helped Arlan to fully function for years without an ACL.

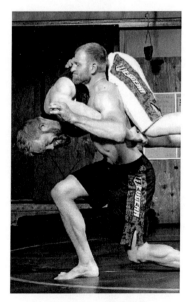

A strong core is essential to protecting your lumbar spine while under load.

stabilized the joint enough for him to continue his extremely active lifestyle.

Stronger bodies are more resilient and more resistant to injuries. Many of the overuse injuries I see in my massage practice can be remedied by general strength training. Weak gluteals and core often lead to low back pain. Shoulder pain is frequently the result of weak upper back and external rotators. Knee pain can be the result of weak hamstrings. A weak body, under load, can suffer from a lot of issues. It is also important to note however that strong bodies that don't move well (poor mobility) can also be susceptible to problems. There always needs to be balance.

At a specific anatomical strength level, we find the core to be of utmost importance. World-renowned strength coach and 5-time UK National Taekwondo champion Alwyn Cosgrove tells the story, "I got hit in the spine once during a taekwondo match. Funny thing is he went through my stomach and rib cage to do it. I got real interested in core training after that." An athlete with a weak core is always at a disadvantage and also has a greater potential for injury. For a soldier, often carrying huge loads, a weak core frequently leads to an eventual back injury.

For our interpretation of the word, core means not only the abdominal and low back region, though they are certainly a vital part of it. Core to us means everything but the extremities. In his book, *Core Performance*, Mark Verstegen calls this "pillar" strength. True abdominal strength is undeniably important, but so is hip strength. So is shoulder stability. Without a complete strong core, everything we do with our extremities puts them at great risk, and nearly guarantees our shoulders and backs will be injured. Core work will not be limited to specific abdominal exercises, but will include any exercise where the spine is stabilized by bracing of the surrounding musculature. Dead-lifts are a core exercise. Squats are a core exercise. Push-ups are a core exercise. They will be used extensively, as will many of the exercises in my first book, *Warrior Core: Core Training Secrets for the Modern Combat Athlete.*

We also see superb grip strength as essential. In

grappling, the fighter with greater grip strength, and the ability to use that strength, will be able to control his opponent to a much greater degree. I'm sure many of you have occasionally rolled with guys who controlled you so well with their grip that you were essentially helpless, unable to escape or attack. In addition to grappling, grip strength will help you in virtually every other area of strength training as well; from pull-ups, to bench press, to dead-lifts (this being said, we will not be using wrist straps to dead-lift!). In his book *Mastering the Twister*, Eddie Bravo explains that he favors squeeze strength to grip strength. While I still feel grip strength is more important, squeeze strength is also very important – especially for MMA, but really for any kind of hand-to-hand combat. We train for both.

In his book *Lone Survivor*, Marcus Luttrell tells of 4 SEALs repeatedly falling down the side of a mountain crashing through trees, rocks, and over cliffs while being pursued by the Taliban. Somehow, their weapons stayed with them. Marcus would stop his fall and his rifle would be within a couple feet of him. I've tripped on a rock in the trail and dropped my water bottle. How do you keep a rifle with you while tumbling head over heals down 900 feet of steep, rough mountain terrain? I'm willing to bet good grip helps. The knowledge that your weapon is likely all that stands between you and the enemy also helps. For those who use firearms at all, grip is of utmost importance. Working with Randy Watt, our fitness priorities for shooting accuracy are leg strength, core strength, and grip strength.

Endurance

Many people equate endurance to running. Certainly this is a way to train for endurance, as are other forms of aerobic exercise. When my primary priority is durability however, I will focus less on running and more on high repetition strength training. Rucking and load carries will also be used consistently. For the soldier, distance running is essential as it is part of the PT test. It can also be beneficial in terms of cardiovascular fitness and muscular endurance, but I definitely feel it is over-used. To quote Frank Palkoska again, during the presentation I attended, he pointed out, "If I ever have to run two miles in battle, something went horribly wrong!" As Mogadishu proved, sometimes things do go horribly wrong, so it is good to be prepared.

Additionally, as a sports massage therapist and sports injury specialist, nearly 75% of injuries I see are running related. IT band syndrome, runner's knee, plantar fasciitis, shin splints, trochanteric bursitis, SI joint issues, and low back and hip pain all are relatively easily prevented overuse issues I see on nearly a daily basis. We should still run, but Battle Tested will revamp your running schedule to give you superior results while running less.

For the fighter, endurance and conditioning are often synonymous. Conditioning is the ability of an MMA athlete to go three to five rounds without burning out. It doesn't matter how strong, how fast, or how technical an athlete is if they are completely spent in the second round. Fighters must be able to protect themselves, and keep coming at their opponent for the duration of the competition. That is conditioning. That is endurance.

People tend to focus on aerobic endurance or "cardio." In all honesty, the parts of combat that matter most are anaerobic and muscular endurance. We will train primarily to improve these. But you know what? Your aerobic endurance will get better too. For years I tested the mile run in my group fitness classes. In an 8-week class, we would run a mile at the beginning for a baseline and run again after eight weeks. Through circuit training, improving strength, and high repetition work, everyone's mile time improved without even running!

Speed/Power/Agility

Speed, power, and agility are all very positive and desirable attributes of the combat athlete. We will absolutely pursue and develop each of these aspects of fitness in the Battle Tested program; however, they are secondary to durability. The fastest athletes, the most explosive, and the most agile, are not always the most durable. It is better for us to focus first on mobility, strength (both of which will help speed, power, and agility), and endurance to build the resilience we need to stay in the fight.

Chaos

Battle is chaotic. Training for chaos is crucial. Regardless of how much you have trained, how much you have prepared, anything could happen. There is a well known Mike Tyson quote, *"Everyone has a plan until they get punched in the mouth"*. Whether in battle or competition, we can plan and prepare for the big picture of what the opponent will likely do, but once engaged in combat, the real-time fight is highly unpredictable. Second-by-second, anything can happen. Knowing this, we need to be aware in our training that it isn't always going to be pre-determined, carefully planned sets and repetitions. We need to deliberately incorporate chaos, both unpredictability and technical skills in high stress, high intensity environments.

I was at a National Strength and Conditioning Association conference attending a hands-on session by Institute of Human Performance founder Juan Carlos Santana. 160 people all did a circuit together with resistance bands, medicine balls, and speed ladders. With a pile of assorted equipment in the middle of the room, Santana had half of the group come to the middle and grab something, then return to our spot circling the room. From there we set up our equipment, grabbed a partner and begin circling the room, spending 30 seconds going all out on the exercise then taking 15 seconds to move to the next piece of equipment. Frequently we would end up going from all out on one exercise for 30 seconds to the very same exercise again.

Santana made it a point that the real world is like that. You are not going to be in the middle of a title fight, or in the middle of a firefight and be able to take a break and work a different muscle group because you legs are spent or your lungs are screaming. You need to be able to suck it up and push through whatever comes up.

In July 2011, Juan Carlos Santana wrote in an article on functional training,

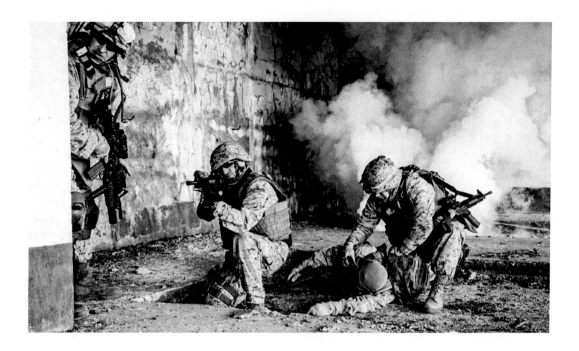

"Eventually integrate a significant amount of controlled chaos into the training. Sports, and life in general, are chaotic and unstable in nature. The more chaos an individual rehearses, the better they will react under unrehearsed-play conditions." With this viewpoint, we will be utilizing various methods of training to incorporate chaos and unpredictability into our workouts.

In addition to performing random unpredictable activities, chaos in battle also requires performing technical skills in less than ideal environments, while fatigued, or with your heart beating out of your chest. In Natural Born Heroes, McDougall makes the point, "Because that's the ugly truth about heroism: the tests don't start when you're ready or stop when you are tired. You don't get time-outs, warm-ups, or bathroom breaks. You may have a headache or be wearing the wrong pants or find yourself – the way Norina did – in a skirt and low heels in a school hallway becoming slick with your own blood." Now most of you probably don't wear skirts or heels, but you get the point. McDougall also describes the reality of life for Resistance fighters on the island of Crete during WWII, "Xan had been on the move for nearly two full days by that point and eaten little more than bread crusts, but rested or exhausted, fed or famished, go-time for a guerrilla is non-negotiable."

I frequently hear people at both at the gym and at martial arts schools making excuses for poor performance or lack of energy. They avoid certain things because they already lifted early that morning, or they are sore from yesterday's chest workout. Given similar skill level, I'm confident I will beat that person nearly every time. If you are a warrior, you need to understand that the battle doesn't wait for the conditions all to be right. I like what strongman Arthur Saxon said in 1905, "The man who can miss a night's rest or miss a meal or two without showing any ill effect or without losing any physical power, is better entitled to be considered a strong man than the man who is only apparently strong, being possessed of momentary strength, which is, after all, a muscle test pure and simple."

I expect warriors to be ready always, regardless of how much they squatted the day before. I frequently have interns from the local university who spend a semester at my gym. We naturally encourage them to jump in with us whatever we are doing. It is interesting to see the difference in response. Most are strong, capable, athletic individuals, but only some are willing to join in, regardless of their weekly lifting regimen. While it is true that there are physiological benefits to meticulous programming and carefully planned out rest days, etc. - the mental edge from being willing to throw down anytime is more important and will serve you better in battle. Powerlifting icon Louie Simmons says, "It is easy to train in order to be the best on the best day possible. Do NOT fall for this trap. You must train to be the best on the worst day possible!!"

On November 2, 2017, I attempted to set a new Guinness World Record (GWR) for 'Most Squat Thrusts in 1 minute while wearing a 100 lb. backpack'. A strap on my pack broke on my first repetition and 100 lbs smashed me in the back of the head on it's way to the floor. The current record was 13 repetitions in 1 minute, and we joked that, "At least it didn't happen on rep 12!" We quickly transferred the weight to another pack and started again. On the 13th repetition the waist belt broke. Knowing I couldn't stop, I kept going only to have the arm strap of a second pack tear off and the weight once again smash me in the back of the head on what would have been the record rep. We took a break to rest, eat and run home for a better backpack, and planned to meet up in few hours for another attempt. The situation was far from ideal. My neck hurt, my low back hurt, and my legs were completely smoked. It was getting late and I had been up since 4am. Not only that, two of the required independent witnesses to the attempt were unable to come back later, so we were scrambling to find new witnesses that could and would come with minimal notice. Returning to the gym three hours later I was slightly concerned I might be too beat up to surpass the 13 repetition record. Just before 11pm, I hit 15 repetitions in 1 minute. Six months later GWR disqualified my attempt because I didn't reach complete hip extension at the bottom of each repetition. You win some, you lose some. Nevertheless, it was a learning experience and a good opportunity to push through when things go wrong and learn from my mistakes.

Training in chaos could be firearm training mixed with high intensity exercises (look up Pat McNamara on YouTube - you won't regret it), pre-fatigued hand-to-hand techniques, card workouts where you randomly draw your number of reps, or circuits where a partner calls out what exercise you will do next. A little bit about blending technical training with strength and conditioning. I frequently hear people say what a horrible idea it is to do conditioning before skills training. Being tired will negatively affect technique, etc, etc. Maybe so, but in my experience, well-matched opponents rarely get submitted when they are fresh and battles during war aren't always going to wait until you're well rested. Rather

MMA fights frequently end when one fighter gets tired, defense gets sloppy, and the better-conditioned athlete pushes the pace and begins to take control of the situation.

I really like a quote I saw by Brazilian Jiu-Jitsu world champion Caio Terra on training technique, "Train to do things without energy and make the technique good. Otherwise you will learn that the move only works when you're in shape or have energy. That is not a good technique. By learning the proper technique, you'll find when you are really tired, have nothing left, and you're in a match and start to wonder 'What is my salvation?' you will know you can do the move with no energy left. Technique is your salvation." If you're technique only works when you are not tired, you will have a hard time being successful as a competitor.

By conditioning before skill training, you learn to rely on technique. For years, one of our guys went to Jiu-Jitsu class straight from our toughest training day. He is an absolute monster and intentionally did it to neutralize his strength advantage at class and force himself to rely on technique. His technique flourished. When training for occasional long races, I try to schedule trail runs immediately prior to Jiu-Jitsu class. I love showing up to class pre-fatigued, never sure if my professor will choose today to push conditioning hard.

We lost a great soldier, friend and training partner, Miles Vigil, on November 29th, 2010. A former collegiate football player and Army veteran, Miles was a straight-up beast, weighing in at around 265 and strong as an ox. Sparring with him, you expected to get absolutely crushed, run over by a bigger, stronger man. The surprising thing was that Miles was one of the more technical Jiu-Jitsu guys I have trained with. Everything he did was so technical that you never felt how big he was. I strive to be like Miles on the mat, and conditioning before I train Jiu-Jitsu helps.

Hand-to-Hand Combat

There is something about actually going toe-to-toe with another human that is both invigorating, eye opening, and absolutely necessary. The website, The Onion, posted a YouTube video in 2014 reporting that men were on average 4,000% less effective in fights than they imagine (https://www.youtube.com/watch?v=fe3na9umxDA). It is obviously hilarious satire, but likely holds more truth than most men would like to admit. Men constantly mentally weigh themselves against other guys and imagine scenarios in their head of what they would do if it came to contact. Again, "*Everyone has a plan until they get punched in the mouth*". This is known as the Dunning-Kruger Effect. In a nutshell, incompetent people grossly over-estimate their competence. This happens with fighting, but can happen in any segment of the Survival Readiness Triangle. Many people think they have their mental game together. Many people think they are stronger, faster, and more fit than average. Many people think they would know what to do in a life-or-death situation. The fascinating thing about the Dunning-Kruger Effect is that the ONLY way to realize you are incompetent is to learn the skill, and reflect on what your skill level "used" to be. What are

YOU lacking? Be honest with yourself and make a decision NOW to focus on improving your weakness. If hand-to-hand combat is not part of your training and you face someone who knows what they are doing, when it matters, you WILL lose.

Participating in martial arts allows you to learn more about yourself. In Jiu-Jitsu we say, "*You can't hide on the mat*." Regardless of how big a man acts, how loud he talks, or how much he thinks of himself, when it comes to sparring, there is nowhere to hide how effective or un-effective he actually is. Most of you are either fighters or have some experience with military combatives, so you have an idea how you stack up. You also know, it is often the soft-spoken, scrawny guy with cauliflower ear that you have to watch out for.

If you haven't trained in martial arts, start immediately. Train frequently and train consistently. You can never train too much for a job that can kill you. Agent T from *Order in Chaos* in chapter 1, credits his martial arts training with making him a more effective police officer. He explains, "Since I started training in Jiu-Jitsu, my physical altercations with other people in the job have reduced dramatically. And that's a confidence thing on my part, and it's also knowing the realities. I don't want to get hurt. I don't want to fight this guy. What can I do to solve this without fighting? And I credit that to Jiu-Jitsu 100%. That is what separates Jiu-Jitsu from the lifting."

In terms of physical preparation, combat is much different than any other exercise. Whether kickboxing, grappling, or fighting MMA, combat is exhausting. Nothing can prepare you for fighting like actual fighting. Controversial though he may be, I love what SEAL Team Six founder Richard Marcinko says about physical contact in his book Rogue Warrior:

> "We hiked. We camped. We shot the hell out of targets. When we had time, we'd waltz into Virginia Beach for some full-contact bar-brawling.
> A word or two here about that. I have always believed that being a SEAL, like being an NFL linebacker, requires a certain amount of aggressive, close physical contact with your fellow human beings. Some may disagree with me. But I find there is something truly rewarding about putting your back up against the back of someone you trust with your life, and taking on all comers. Sure, you take a certain number of dings in the pursuit of these unruly activities. But in the long run, I believe the rewards outweigh the liabilities. And when, as an officer, my most important job is to build unit integrity, there are few better ways in which to build it than late at night, in a bar, when it's you and your five guys against the rest of the world."

Now from a fitness and performance standpoint, I can't promote late nights at the bar, but Marcinko is preaching physical contact, testing yourself against others. And while the bar might not be the best place to do that, tournaments (whether grappling, judo, kickboxing, etc.) are a suitable substitute. Marcinko's point about team unity is spot on too. Nothing builds team unity like training, then fighting together.

IMMEDIATE ACTION #2

<u>Recruit a Battle Buddy</u>

It is possible to follow the program in this book by yourself. That being said, it will be much easier to do it with a friend or teammate. It is infinitely easier to get out of bed in the morning, or head to the gym after a long day at work if you know someone is waiting for you there. And not just any friend, but a friend who will hold you accountable and not let you slack off. You need a buddy that you absolutely don't want to let down. You need a buddy who won't let you down either - who is dependable, committed, and won't let you back out.

Make a list right now of five people who might be a good fit. Commit to contacting them one by one this week until one of them agrees to training three days a week with you. Beyond the obvious accountability of having a workout partner, there are many exercises in this book that require a partner. There are exercises you can replace them with if you don't have a partner, but you would be missing out on part of what makes this book great.

Make your list here and start your selection process.

1 _____

2 _____

3 _____

4 _____

5 _____

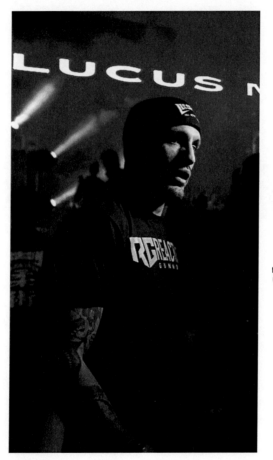

Chapter 3
The Power of the Mind

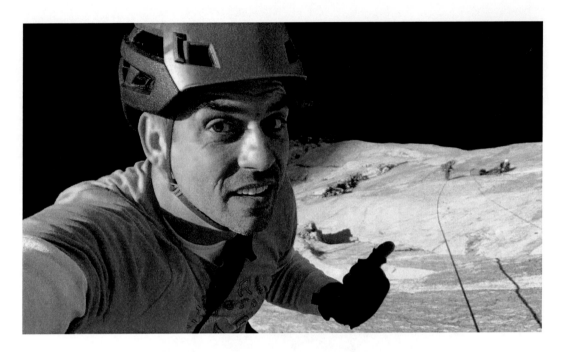

Chapter 3 – The Power of the Mind

"There comes a time when preparation no longer counts. I know that ultimately not how quickly I can tie knots that will make the difference, but rather how strong my heart is – how much I really want this, how much I will be able to endure up there. It is the spirit that counts for everything. I pray that mine will be strong."
                    -Bear Grylls diary entry May 7, 1998 while climbing Mt. Everest

The company IronMind, used to sell a couple great shirts which said: "*A lot of physical is mental.*" and "*10 + willpower = 20*". Mental strength and endurance are even a greater need than physical strength and endurance. It takes quite a bit of mental preparation just to step into the ring with someone whose number one goal is to hurt you enough that you can't continue the fight. Likewise, mental strength is more important to special warfare guys than physical strength. That is why programs for SEALs, Rangers, PJs, Green Berets, etc., go to such great lengths to force people to quit. People who go into the program are already in great shape and believe they have what it takes to survive.

In his book *The Finishing School,* former SEAL Dick Couch explains, "Most of these men are physically capable, but they lack the mental toughness to continue. Most still want to be Navy SEALs. They simply didn't understand the price of admission to this club." This is important to note. Everyone who enters special operations programs has likely already achieved exceptional fitness, and believes that they can persevere and do what it takes.

The instructors want the program to be so difficult and miserable that they break people's will to continue. They want to see who will quit when things get unbearable, and who would rather die trying than give up. Doing whatever it takes to accomplish the mission, long after the physical body begins to fail is what sets Special Operators apart, it's what makes them the most elite soldiers in the world. In his book *The Fighter's Mind*, Sam Sheridan tells of interviewing the army psychologists at Fort Bragg, NC about mental toughness. "I asked about teaching mental toughness – if that was part of Special Forces training the answer was an amused, 'No.' The men who were there had learned it already, somewhere else. They battled their way through training on their own. Their mental toughness skills had to be proved before they even got to this point – not taught to them now."

In his the postscript of his book *SAS Survival Handbook*, John 'Lofty' Wiseman, 26 year veteran of the elite British Special Air Service writes, "Survival is as much a mental attitude as physical endurance and knowledge. Think of survival skills as a pyramid, built on the foundation of that will to survive. People with it have survived even though they did everything against the rule book." In the same way, frequently the people you look at and think they are perfect human specimens with everything it takes to be successful in combat, are the first to wash out when the going gets tough. Most special operators are not the biggest, strongest, most intimidating candidates. Rather they are simply men who refuse to quit.

Plan for Success

It is necessary to be mentally ready BEFORE you get to selection or you are not going to make the cut. It is necessary to be mentally prepared before a fight or tournament, or you may easily lose to a fighter less talented. You need to make a conscious decision to succeed. You can't go into a pursuit with the thought, "I think I can do this!" Success demands commitment. In his well-known book *The Art of War*, ancient Chinese general, Sun Tzu, writes, "Every battle is won before it is ever fought." What people don't always realize is that every battle is also lost before it is ever fought. If you do not commit 100% to succeed and plan appropriately, you will fail in any great pursuit.

At a submission only grappling tournament in April 2011, I made the heavyweight nogi finals. When asked when I was up next, I replied, "I'm fighting for 1st or 2nd right now." Fighter and friend Jason South, quickly replied, "No. You are fighting for 1st." I had lost perspective. Subconsciously, I had already accepted that I might not win. I eventually did lose a 20-minute battle, but the lesson will stick with me forever. I'm always fighting for 1st.

Sometimes in competition, it is easy to lose sight of the goal. You may be outmatched, exhausted, or behind on points, whatever. But as soon as you concede that you might not win, you have lost. Looking at the opponent, or bracket full of opponents you have to get through in a tournament, it is easy to lose sight that you are fighting for first. A couple years ago I started doing a little mental drill everywhere I competed. I call it *Find the 'Ones'*. It is a constant reminder of the goal in any setting. I spend five to ten minutes looking around the venue, focusing on the goal prior to competition, but can also revisit it at any time during the event. Here's how it works:

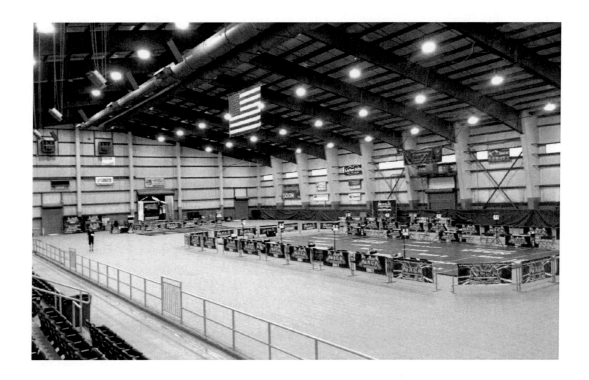

IMMEDIATE ACTION #3
Find The 'Ones'

This is a photo of the venue I competed in at a 2016 grappling tournament.
Look at it closely and find the 'ones'. Every vertical line is a visual
reminder that **I am in it for 1st place**.

The best part is that I am the only one who sees them. The only person in the venue
who is literally surrounded by my goal by the thousands! Look around yourself now.
Wherever you are, they are there, thousands of ones. Seeing them is the secret. It is
a huge mental advantage for me, and can be for you. Just looking around I can't help
but smile, knowing that I am prepared for battle. Not just to compete, but to win. My
opponents have no idea that I am essentially competing INSIDE my vision board.
That is powerful. Do I always win? Of course I don't. Do I fight like I'm going to?
Absolutely!

Find Your Why

The first step in planning for success is to identify WHY you want to succeed. If your why is not strong enough, you will fold when the going gets tough. In The Strength Psychology Instruction Manual, Mike Gillette tells us, "Without a clear commitment to fight, you probably won't. It's too painful and requires too much energy." You need to commit. You need to find your reason, your motivation and define why it is important to you. Then commit. Any reason can be a successful why if it is strong enough. Sometimes it is simply the desire to be the best. Sometimes the goal is a lifelong dream, a goal you've known since childhood that you were meant to pursue. Sometimes it is to prove doubters wrong. I am often motivated by the thought that something can't be done.

A client I helped prepare to climb Everest wanted to know if she was mentally strong enough. Twice she had gone to Nepal to climb, only to be denied by the worst disasters the mountain has ever seen (2014 avalanche in the icefall, and 2015 earthquake caused avalanche through base camp). Yet she returned. She knew it would be painful, but knew that she was physically strong enough. What she didn't know is if she would be able to continue when voices in her head started telling her to turn around. That question was her "why" and it haunted her until she stood at 29,035 feet on May 23, 2017.

Whatever your motivation, make sure it is strong enough to keep you going when your entire being begs for you to quit. In Kiss or Kill, Mark Twight tells of Canadian climber Kevin Doyle. "The first day we climbed 3,000 vertical feet. Day two we put the hammer down and did another 5,000. It started to hurt. Some people chase pain harder than others, consciously or subconsciously. Some use it to inflate their sense of self-importance. Others test their will by working through it. Each of us has a threshold someplace short of serious harm. Kevin's different. His definition of pain is more highly evolved than others. He's willing to hurt himself permanently to get what he wants. In a conversation about calories, he told me that there is always something left to burn, 'even if it's brain matter.' Kevin is, without question, the best I've ever seen. From watching him, I learned to overcome myself." Whatever the "why", Kevin is committed. I wouldn't want to face a man like Kevin Doyle in any battle.

Determination – Get Comfortable Being Uncomfortable

Comfort is a funny thing. Throughout life, we learn to pursue comfort and technology that makes life easier, then, bust our butts in the gym trying to negate the effects comfort and technology have on our body. In his book What Doesn't Kill Us, Scott Carney, who initially set out to write a book debunking The Iceman, Wim Hof, writes, "There is one thing that we do know, however: The invention of technology, as a rule, seems to correlate with a general weakening of the raw physicality and resilience of our species." One thing successful warriors understand is that growth happens outside of your comfort zone. Not only does the physical body benefit, living outside your comfort zone challenges your mind and helps you adapt to adverse situations.

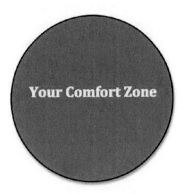

**Where The
Magic Happens**

A well designed strength and conditioning program can be a great way to venture outside your comfort zone. It is easy to do the things you enjoy however, or to focus on your strengths. The key is doing the things you don't want to do. I love what 4-time world heavyweight boxing champion, Evander Holyfield, says in his autobiography, *Becoming Holyfield*, about training for what he considers his greatest fight of all time against Dwight Muhammad Qawi, "Part of that kind of conditioning is obviously to try and improve your stamina, but the other part, and just as important, is to get you familiar with being exhausted so you learn in advance how to deal with it and it doesn't surprise and shock you when it happens."

This is how to create success. This is where champions, and elite soldiers are made. Who can continue to fight long after their physical body has nothing left? When designing workouts for my combat guys, I consciously think, "What don't I want to do? If I was going to do this exercise, how many would I do, or how long would I go?" That is my baseline. I then raise the difficulty above baseline and that's what we do. Once I tell my athletes the goal, I myself am committed too. Chances are pretty good that while I may want desperately to quit, so does everyone else. But none of us will be the first to give up, so we all suffer through together, encouraging and motivating each other along the way.

I once carried a 113-pound rock up and over a mountain through the snow on a winter camping trip (https://www.youtube.com/watch?v=K82eB2pr5z8). Nearly everyone who heard the story asked, "Why?" In all honesty, I did it simply to see if I could. The same was true when I progressed from the 335 lb. tires we frequently flip to a 1,250 lb. beast that barely fit in the UHAUL truck. Why? Again, just to see if I could do it. There is tremendous satisfaction, and huge confidence gain in doing things most other people won't even try, just because you feel like it. In his manual, Mike Gillete says the following:

Remind Yourself to <u>Love</u> the Struggle
Love the process, the fight, the breakthroughs and the struggles. Loving to win is easy. Loving the process moves you to a whole new level of skill. Loving the battle happens because you make it happe**n.**

Typically, the most successful competitors are those who are putting in hard work when others are taking a break. For about a year in college, I had a roommate, Joe Wilson, who was a Division 1 All-American runner. He also won both the Ogden and St. George Marathons (both Boston qualifiers) in the same year shortly after finishing his running career at Weber State University. The year I lived with him, he would race 5Ks and 10Ks and finish 3-5 minutes before the 2nd place runner. I interviewed Joe shortly after he won the St. George Marathon. Joe had a great perspective to putting in the effort. "I love to run in the snow, because I know that most people aren't."

I've adopted a similar approach to fitness in general. Much of what we do, we do specifically because few other people, if any, are doing it. Most people shake their heads when they hear some of the things my friends and I have done to challenge ourselves. The truth is, many people are capable of doing the things we have done, but they sound absurd enough that few will ever try. And when the snow is flying, don't be surprised to find us outside doing farmer walks, speed work, or distance running (Which I despise, of course. Doing it in nasty weather actually makes it much more enjoyable for me).

Doing things the hard way, embracing the suck, goes a long way in the pursuit of success. In his 2008 documentary, *Strong*, well known collegiate and NFL football strength coach, Joe DeFranco explains, "You line up next to a guy, he might be a great athlete, but you think about how you train, you know you're lifting heavy chains, all these heavy bands, and all these awkward objects, and flipping tires, that's a huge mental edge. The physical strength that you gain from this type of program is awesome, but the mental edge to know that the guy standing across from you has no idea the type of training we do, nor could he go through that, that might be more important, more beneficial than the physical strength that goes with this program".

Look at most successful people and you will see a common theme. They are determined and not afraid of hard work. In his book Iceman – My Fighting Life, Chuck Liddell tells of a challenge with his high school wrestling coach who competed in the local police league, "If I won, the entire team could take off that day's conditioning drills; if he won, we had to do double the work: an extra set of sprints, an extra set of rope climbs, an extra round of wrestling without breaks. Everyone always felt sick to their stomachs after one round of conditioning drills. Two would have been brutal. Then I pinned the coach in the first round, and while all my teammates were cheering, I yelled, 'Screw it, we're doing the drills.' That's how I was winning, and being in that good of shape didn't come easy."

In addition to being willing to do the work, success is built on not quitting when the work seems unbearable. Everyone always has at least a little more that they can give. More than they think they are able to. People who realize that, embrace it, and challenge themselves to keep going, are warriors that will be hard to outperform on the battlefield.

Self Awareness

Self-awareness is the foundation for being able to respond to any other emotion. You are going to have anxiety or other emotional reactions before a fight. Being self-aware helps you process these emotions and act accordingly. Self-awareness is being confident. But it is also about being aware of your limitations. I'm not saying you shouldn't strive to surpass your limitations, by all means you should! Simply know where you are weak and working on those areas is key to rising above your limitations.

Remember the Dunning Kruger Effect? Interestingly, the more competent someone becomes, the more they realize just how much they still have to learn. I know I am a very competent grappler. I also know many people locally who are better than I am. Then there is that next level of grappler that make all of us look like amateurs. I have been training nearly 10 years and have a lifetime still to learn. This is why I don't understand arrogance. With very few exceptions, there is ALWAYS someone better. The guys that obnoxiously let everyone know they are the best around are the guys I most want to test. The difference between confidence and arrogance is silence.

In a February 2017 article in Recoil Magazine, Pat McNamara (www.tmacsinc.com) a former 13-year member of Delta Force explains, "Some time back, I was part of a small group of individuals who had the mindset that there was and there is no second place. It wasn't shouted in some lame mantra nor was there any chest pounding. It's a fundamental mindset that resonates with certain people or groups of people."The best know they don't have to try and convince everyone around them that they are the best. They simply do what they do, and people notice.

While being aware of your weaknesses is vital to progress, being aware of your strengths and preparedness and being confident in your abilities is essential to success. You can't go into a fight focused on your weaknesses and short-comings. You need to be aware of them and act accordingly, confident in your ability to overcome your limitations. In his article *Justification for an Elitist Attitude*, Mark Twight notes the power of the mind, "And despite understanding my humanity, I still feel superior within a narrowly defined discipline. Mostly because I've proven how far a disciplined mind can take the man that isn't particularly strong, or brave." Confidence in battle is part of your plan for success. It is the only way you can win the battle before it is fought.

While confidence itself is a mental state, it is inseparable from the physical. John Danaher, coach behind the famed Danaher Death Squad (a grappling team that includes the likes of Garry Tonon, Gordon Ryan, Eddie Cummings, and Nicky Ryan), explains it like this:

> "Confidence may be a mental attribute, but its birth is physical – the hours, months, and years of training that create superior technique which leads to victory. The first victories will be small, unheralded gym victories, seen by no one other than yourself. As those small victories accumulate they will be replaced by even bigger victories until an unshakable faith in your ability walks within you and people call it confidence. Yes – in its mature form it is a mental attribute, but never forget that its infancy was physical."

Legitimate confidence comes only as a result of intense physical preparation.

Preparation

Knowing that you are better trained, have worked harder, and have been more disciplined goes a long way towards improving confidence. Jock Lewes, the man tasked with physical and mental preparation for the members of the newly formed British SAS, above all, "…sought to make the men so inured to hardship that the reality, when it came, would feel almost easy. 'The confident man will win,' Lewes insisted." This is echoed in the book *Natural Born Heroes*. "The art of the hero wasn't about being brave; it was about being so competent that bravery wasn't an issue." Like confidence, competence can only come from incessant preparation.

On June 3, 2017, Alex Honnold did the unthinkable by free soloing (climbing without ropes or any other safety gear) the 3,000 foot El Capitan in Yosemite. Not only did he become the first climber to free solo El Cap, he took a route called Freerider, a notoriously difficult route that is quite noteworthy when successfully climbed WITH ropes, and completed it in a mere 3 hours and 56 minutes. The only two other soloists who ever publicly admitted considering El Cap, Michael Reardon and Dean Potter, are both dead. Reardon drowned in 2007 after being swept off a sea cliff in Ireland, and Potter died in a base-jumping accident in Yosemite in 2015.

A National Geographic article about the climb explains that Honnold is obsessive about training and "spends hours perfecting, rehearsing and memorizing exact sequences of hand and foot placement for every key pitch. He is an inveterate note-taker, logging his workouts and evaluating his performance on every climb in a detailed journal." In a post-climb interview Alex admits it felt much less scary than other solos he had done. When asked which ones, Alex stated, "Probably all of them. Because I put so much work into this one. I was so dialed. There was no uncertainty on this. I knew exactly what to do the whole way. A lot of the handholds feel like old friends."

In an article for Outside Online, friend and climber Tommy Caldwell said of Alex, "He's climbed the Freerider at least a dozen times and practiced the most difficult sections to the point where he likely would have been able to do them blindfolded. But free soloing is a feat less physical than mental. Beyond the obvious factors of vertigo inducing exposure and

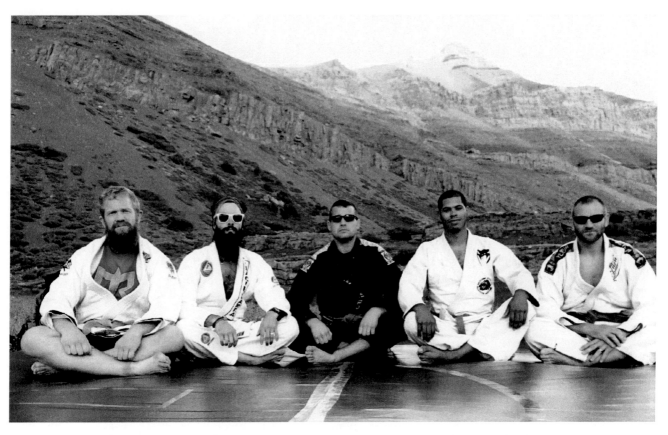

unexpected obstacles (think breaking rock and birds flying out of cracks), hard granite climbing requires such precision that one must be completely lucid."

Be Part of a Team

I have competed in a huge variety of team and individual sports throughout my life. I'm often drawn to individual sports; but even then, I am part of a team. Fellow competitors, training partners, fans, there is always a team behind a successful competitor. Nothing compares to unity you build training and competing with a hard working team. Surround yourself with people you believe in. Surround yourself with people that will make you better. Surround yourself with people who will not settle for anything less than your best. It is easy to disappoint yourself, then justify your actions or lack of action. It is harder to know you are letting others down. Surround yourself with training partners and teammates that will not accept mediocrity. Surround yourself with people you would trust your life with. And here's the kicker - people you would GIVE your life for.

Lasting bonds form quickly while suffering. When you go through a challenging training session with someone, there is an immediate connection. A bond stitched together by the shared experience. Knowing you have worked more intimately together than most, that you have pushed yourselves to the limit, without allowing each other to falter, builds trust. This is important to note. As part of a team, you need to do your part. It isn't enough to coast along enjoying the success of the team. If you wish to share trust with a team, it is necessary to do your part. If you aren't contributing to your team, they will look for someone to take your place. Trust works both ways. If you trust your team but they don't trust you to step up when you are needed, you aren't a worthwhile member of the team. But when you put in the effort to build that mutual trust, a team is a powerful thing.

In Band of Brothers, Ambrose explains, "The result of these shared experiences was a closeness unknown to all outsiders. Comrades are closer than friends, closer than brothers. Their relationship is different from that of lovers. Their trust in, and knowledge of each other is total." He goes on to recount the words of Pvt. Kurt Gabel of the 513th PIR, "'The three of us, Jake, Joe, and I became…an entity. Often three such entities would make up a squad, with incredible results in combat. They would literally insist on going hungry for one another, freezing for one another, dying for one another. And the squad would try to protect them or bail them out without regard to consequences…'"

Competition

Early in my Jiu-Jitsu career, a training partner told me, "You can roll and practice all you like, but tournaments are etched in your mind forever." Interestingly, losing, it seems is etched deeper than winning. I have won tournaments, and in most cases remember the submission I finished my opponent with in the final. The opponents leading up to the final, I remember a few. But I can tell you very little about the rest of the match. My losses though, hurt. I can name the people I have lost to over the years. The most important fights I have lost are burned on my soul. I can play them back moment by moment and tell you exactly what mistakes I made, when I made them, and what the consequences were.

Competition is essential to progressing in combat sports. In class though, we are all friends, we more or less have learned the same things, we spar frequently enough to get a feel for each other's strategies, and we aren't really trying to hurt each other. Competition takes it to another level. You often have no idea who your opponent is, what his go-to moves are, how he sets them up, and how he'll defend against your game. And occasionally, he really doesn't mind if he hurts you, he wants to win at all costs. The game changes here, and you really see how you respond to being put in a near real-life situation in which you have to defend yourself. Your opponents' single focus is to win at all costs by causing you enough pain that you give up. The atmosphere of a tournament, the pre-competition butterflies, the adrenaline dump and subsequent fatigue are all game changers. If you are not familiar with these feelings, you could be in trouble when it matters. Competition forces you to deal with these issue BEFORE your life depends on it.

For soldiers, competition is a good chance to see how you do in combat. Training is one thing, but how do you react to someone really trying to hurt you? If I knew I could get called to war at any time, I would spend as much time as I could training, but to take it further, competing any chance I could. Competitive fighting is of course very different from actual combat where you win or die. It is a world of difference and I hesitate to compare it even remotely to war, but competition does give you a feel for how you or someone else will react in combat.

Resilience – Dealing with Adversity

Assuming you are determined and confident, what happens when things don't go your way? You are not always going to win. You will experience lost battles, injuries, family issues, and other setbacks. That is all part of life. How you react to this adversity will determine your effectiveness as a warrior. Louie Simmons says, "Don't be afraid to fail or look like a fool. These are necessary milestones on your way to the top."

Remember Your "Why"

Remember how important it was to find your "why"? When things get tough, you need this to fall back on. What is it that is your driving force? Remembering this can keep you going when you no longer want to. When adversity hits, when you are challenged and your goals start to seem less important, you need to revisit why you set the goals in the first place. If your "why" isn't important enough, you will likely fail when things get hard. Choose your "why" wisely. If you don't have a good enough reason to pursue your goals, you should probably set different goals. If you do have a good enough reason, dwelling on this reason can help you push through difficult circumstances.

Big Picture Mentality

It is easy in the moment to get caught up in how bad we perceive things to be. Chances are you've been through worse. And you survived. You are still here. Maybe you haven't been through worse. Maybe you truly are in the worst possible situation you could be in right now. Assuming you make it through, how important will this moment be when you look back on it five years from now. Will it seem like as big of a deal in the long run as it does right now? Perhaps, but likely not. Depending on the severity of the situation, years from now, you may realize that the current adversity you are facing did indeed have a profound impact on your life. Chances are, your life was changed in some way. Struggles shape our lives and make us who we are. Whether we like it or not, we learn and we grow through adversity. Suffering is an essential part of life. Without suffering, there would be no fear. Without fear, there could be no courage.

Musician Tim Timmons, when diagnosed with terminal cancer 15 years ago said, "The gift of cancer is the gift of perspective." Adversity forces perspective. When faced with death, the important things in life become crystal clear. I saw this in my father's life during his 10 year battle with Non-Hodgkins Lymphoma (likely caused by Agent Orange exposure during the Vietnam War). When faced with death, he spent more time with God, and he spent more time with family. When he passed away, it was devastating, even though we knew it was coming. It was the hardest thing I'd been through, bar none. But I knew without a doubt what was important to him.

In 2016, my daughter, who was 1 year-old at the time, was life-flighted twice for unexplainable complex seizures that could not be stopped. Two times, I watched as the doctors surrounded her trying to stabilize her enough to be loaded on the helicopter and flown to the nearest children's hospital. During those moments, and the following days, sleeping in her hospital room, the important things were clear. My job didn't matter. My hobbies didn't matter. Fitness didn't matter. What mattered was my little girl. What mattered was my trust that she was in God's care. I believe whole-heartedly in a God who created the entire universe, and who also cares for me, and cares for each of us . In the book of Matthew, we read, "Are not two sparrows sold for a penny? Yet not one of them will fall to the ground outside of your Father's care. And even the very hairs of your head are all numbered. So don't be afraid; you are worth more than many sparrows," (Matthew 10:29-31). Even in death, belief in God means that my time on this earth is a minuscule part of his plan. I have comfort knowing whatever happens here on earth, I will live with Him forever in eternity.

Want to hear something else crazy? The Bible actually says that suffering is a good thing! Most of us agree that suffering produces growth, and Romans 5:3-5 confirms this. "Not only so, but we also glory in our sufferings, because we know that suffering produces perseverance; perseverance, character; and character, hope. And hope does not put us to shame, because God's love has been poured out into our hearts through the Holy Spirit, who has been given to us." Philippians 1:29 tells us, "For it has been granted to you on behalf of Christ, not only to believe in him, but also to suffer for him." Then in 1 Peter 4:12-13, Peter

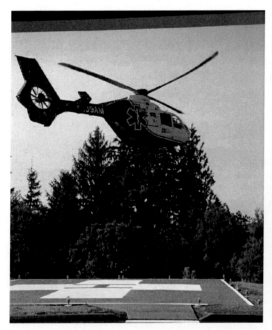

Akia, en route to St. Mary's Children's Hospital in Tacoma, WA. We were driving the Pacific coast out of cell service and just happened to stop for lunch 4 miles from a small hospital.

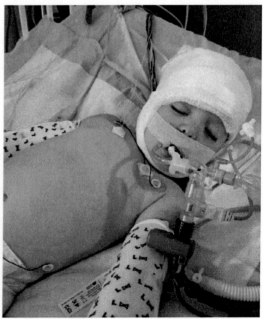

After her second seizure, we didn't see Akia conscious for several days while the doctors ran test after test on her.

writes, "Dear friends, do not be surprised at the fiery ordeal that has come on you to test you, as though something strange were happening to you. But rejoice in as much as you participate in the sufferings of Christ, so that you may be overjoyed when his glory is revealed.

If you don't believe in God, the purpose of this book is not to change your mind, or push my beliefs on you. But it is important to point out that to those who believe, their belief in God makes adversity smaller and more manageable as they have hope in a bigger picture.

Humor

Did you know that laughter is actually proven to elevate pain threshold? In 2011, an article called *Social Laughter is Correlated with an Elevated Pain Threshold* was published in the Proceedings of the Royal Society B. It was based on a series of six experimental studies in both laboratory and natural settings using change in pain as an assay for endorphin release. The authors suggest the significant increase in pain threshold is a result of the physical result of laughing which in turn triggers activation of the endorphin system. Pretty cool, right? Perhaps laughter truly is the best medicine. Sometimes you just have to look at the situation, and laugh. You could cry, and sometimes that is okay too. You could get all pissed off and rant about how much life sucks and refuse to be happy. Or, you can take it in stride, knowing that life is full of ups and downs for everyone; and it is your turn. James Lawrence, The Iron Cowboy, blew everybody's mind in 2015 when he successfully completed 50 Ironman triathlons in 50 days in 50 states. As you might expect, the endeavor was plagued with injury and extreme fatigue and filled with times when he physically and mentally didn't feel like he could go on. In his book, Redefine Possible, James, who also once rode a Ferris wheel for 10 straight days to win $10,000 says, "I have a theory: if you can make a joke, you can take another step."

Optimism

I am a born optimist and worry about very little. This can obviously be good and bad, depending on the situation. When dealing with adversity, however I truly believe this is a necessary quality for optimal performance. A pessimist can likely get through most situations as well (some pessimists are the hardest working, detail oriented people I have ever met) but they will likely grumble their way through, and can demotivate those around them in the process. When faced with difficult situations, you want to be surrounded by encouraging people who give you hope. Hope goes a very long way. Without hope, what do you have to keep you pressing on? When you are hopeful about what can come out of adverse times, and when you are surrounded by an optimistic team, it is easy to work together to make it through.

In The Arena:
Climbing Out of Adversity

April 25, 2015, Ellen woke to a beautiful day at Everest Base Camp (EBC). The sky was a deep, majestic blue; the clouds passing in violent silence over the summit of the world's largest mountain, 12,000 feet above her. She was ready. She had prepared as much as anyone could. Part of this was having a lofty goal, one that she knew left no option for failure. But even more than that, it's simply who she was. It was in her blood, ingrained in her very soul. She was relentless, not willing to quit until she had achieved her goal. Her life revolved around seeing it through. She was fully committed. Committed to the point of resigning her partnership in a busy cardiology clinic two years ago when they didn't want her to come to Everest. Once she quit her job, she dedicated herself to full time training for this climb. In addition to working with a strength coach three days a week, she was doing 6-hour workouts on a bike and climbing up and down various Wasatch mountains with 40 pounds of kitty litter in her backpack, Monster. She had slept for months in an altitude tent and had climbed peaks all over the world. She had done Rainier eight times, Vinson Massif in Antarctica, South America, the Alps, Cho Oyu, and other mountains here in the Himalayas. But it had always been about Everest. All about this moment and the days to come. She had been here before…

One year and seven days earlier, on Good Friday 2014, Ellen woke at 6:30am in her tent to the loudest crash she had ever heard. She quickly unzipped her tent to see a huge plume of ice and snow coming down the west shoulder of Everest. She saw base camp come alive with movement as climbers and support alike, rushed in alarm in search of any way they could help. A physician, Ellen raced to the base camp medical tent, Everest ER, in uncertain anticipation, now in the middle of the biggest single day disaster Everest had ever seen. Once several walking wounded and five critically injured men were stabilized and sent to Kathmandu, Ellen was tasked with taking pictures and trying to identify the Sherpa's as they were long-lined to base camp dangling from a helicopter. In all, 16 Sherpa were killed when an ice block the size of a 10-story building broke free and tumbled down through the Khumbu icefall, destroying and burying everything in its path. 12 victims were recovered that day, another the following day, and 3 will remain buried beneath the ice forever.

Now, a year later, Ellen was reading in her tent when she felt the ground shake violently. At 11:56am Nepal was rocked with a 7.8 magnitude earthquake. The quake triggered an avalanche on the peak opposite the Khumbu Icefall. Ellen unzipped the door of her tent to see the mountainside roaring toward base camp. "I thought I was going to die. I thought, 'This is it, this is the end.'" She immediately hit the deck, knocking a tooth out while diving back into the tent as the air blast preceding the wall of snow and ice flattened everything in its path. When the rumbling and shaking stopped, the middle of base camp had been decimated. Propane tanks, cook stoves, rocks, and other projectiles from the camp had been thrown through EBC by the estimated 250mph blast of air, destroying everything in their path.

Once again, Ellen quickly entered doctor mode. Anyone who could help moved the critically injured down camp, where Ellen and three other doctors began treating the injured in two tents. One tent took long bone fractures and internal injuries and the other tent for head wounds. Ellen worked with another doctor in the head injury tent and within 4-5 hours had 10 men in their care. For the next 18 hours she cared for the injured with the few medical supplies available,. The next morning, courageous helicopter pilots evacuated 60 injured in inclement weather. 22 men had died at EBC, making it now the worst single-day tragedy in Everest history. In Nepal, over 9,000 people had died in the earthquake, and millions were left homeless. Once again, the mountain shut down and the climbing season was over. Ellen returned home again denied a summit attempt by completely uncontrollable circumstances. She came back to horrible nightmares and the thought, "I'm done. I can't do this anymore. I'm not going back."

Fast-forward two years. On May 23, 2017, at -30 degrees, with wind gusts of 80mph, Ellen's 15-year journey was realized as she stood at 29,035 feet. She HAD come back, encouraged by those who believed in her, and not wanting to remember this mountain she loved so dearly as she had left it in 2015. Her summit attempt was not without incident. Five members of her eleven-climber team had left early, unsuccessful. Three climbers had died on May 21st, including one being short-hauled in as Ellen's team arrived at Camp 4. Then, the following day at Camp 4, she was once again called to save lives as a Pakistani climber and his young Sherpa were helped into camp in dire condition. Knowing it could delay or end her own summit bid, Ellen didn't hesitate to offer care.

"For me as a doc, there is no question. The main issue is helping folks when they need help. On a mountain or life in general, it has to be about the larger picture, about helping other people. Because otherwise, I could not feel good about what I accomplished."

Within an hour, the young Sherpa, who seemed sure to die, had completely turned around and was awake and alert. The expedition was still on. With a storm approaching, they left Camp 4 around 10pm. As she reached the South summit, and looked toward the Hillary Step, she started bawling. After so many years and so much effort, she finally realized she was going to do it. By then her team had spread out and she was almost alone. Typically, there are 10-20 people on the summit, but due to the storm, when she arrived at around 6:30am it was Ellen and four others at the top. Her 15-20 minutes at the top of the world were magical and more beautiful than she imagined.

Ellen believes we get where we get in life, when we are supposed to get there. It is necessary in life to embrace one's dream despite what people tell you, then find the people who believe in you.

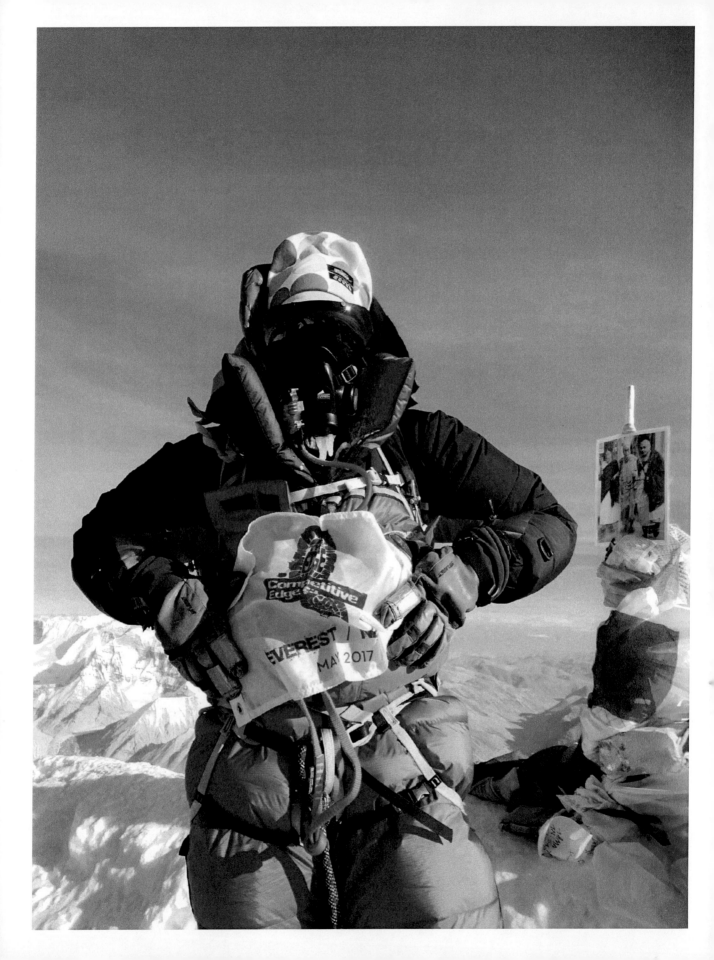

IMMEDIATE ACTION #4
KIMS Test

One quality of a successful warrior is situational awareness; being aware of your surroundings and being able to adapt to the environment and the circumstances. What do you see? What do you need to be wary of? What can you use for your benefit? This is an obviously necessary skill in military and law enforcement, but we also see it in combat sports. Many high level competitors are able to change their strategy on the fly, picking up on their opponents habits and tells, and adapting to use this new information as they learn it to effectively avoid strikes and set up counters.

Variations of the KIMS test are used by various sniper and reconnaissance schools and law enforcement agencies to improve observation and memory. As they repeat the test, they do it under more and more stressful situations and go longer and longer between the observation and when the person tested has to recall what they saw. The test was named after the Ruydyard Kipling book "*Kim*", the story of an Irish orphan, trained as a young man for government intelligence work. How observant are you? How good is your memory? Give this test a try now and let's find out. Here's how it works:

Before you turn the page, set a timer for 60 seconds.

Start the timer and flip the page. For one minute, try to memorize the items in the following picture. When your timer goes off, flip to the next page. You then have 60 seconds to name all of the items in the photo.

Is your timer ready? GO!

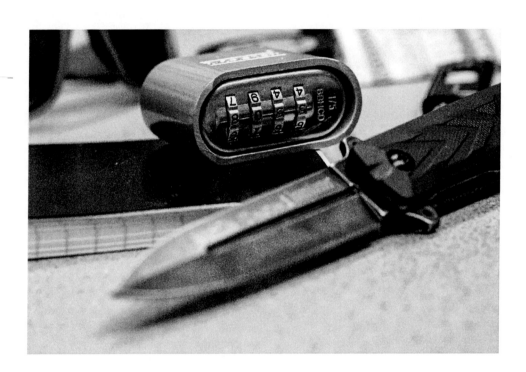

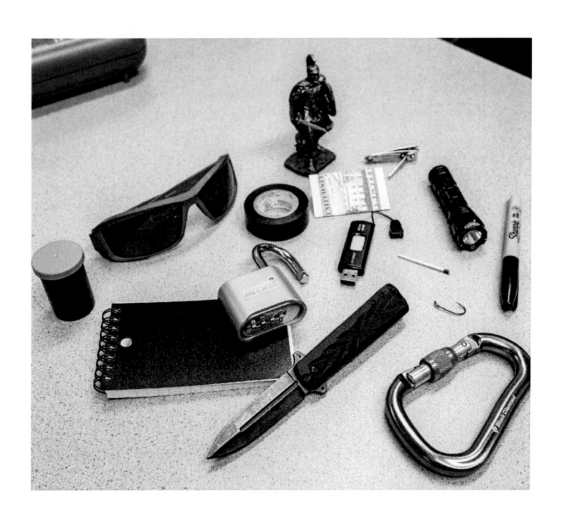

41.226718

You now have 60 seconds to write down as many of the items as you can remember. If you don't finish in 60 seconds, count your items, then keep trying until you simply can't think of any more.

_____

_____

_____

_____

_____

_____

_____

_____

_____

_____

_____

_____

_____

_____

_____

How did you do? Did you remember all 15 items? Did it throw you off that there were 17 lines? Did you know what the film canister was (age test!)?

Now let's see how good you really are.

What was the combination on the Master Lock?

_____   _____   _____   _____

If you didn't see it, look back and memorize it.

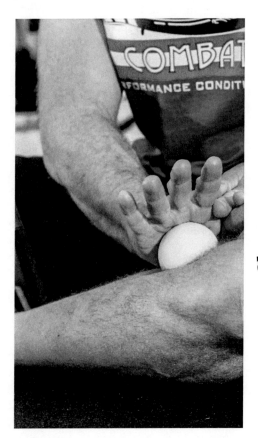

Chapter 4
The Importance of Recovery

Chapter 4 – The Importance of Recovery

Fighters are known for beating their bodies into the ground. Tactical operators are frequently overworked, overloaded and running on minimal sleep. Law enforcement is a notoriously stressful occupation with really weird hours. This is a grey area when planning to implement an intense strength and conditioning program. Where is the line between meeting the demands of the career while improving performance and pushing combat athletes to the point of burnout and injury. MMA fighters are often training Muay Thai, jiu-jitsu, wrestling, and boxing. Occasionally, these various disciplines are taught by the same coach. At higher levels however, fighters often train with multiple specialized coaches, each of whom feel responsible to include conditioning as part of their training. Even without a dedicated strength and conditioning segment, rest and recovery are of utmost importance.

Former UFC fighter and legendary trainer Bobby Maximus (www.bobbymaximus.com), doesn't believe in over-training, only under-recovery. The body is extremely capable of bouncing back from just about anything you subject it to. The issue becomes the amount of time it takes to recover from repeated exhaustive training sessions and the frequency with which you partake in them. If you could destroy yourself physically once a week and spend the rest of the week recovering, it probably wouldn't matter how hard you trained. Unfortunately, it is difficult to improve skill or performance of anything while only training it once a week. Over-training is more an issue of repeated training sessions without allowing proper recovery between sessions. This becomes a very real problem that often shows itself through chronic fatigue and susceptibility to injury. Another clue is resting heart rate. If your resting heart rate is going up instead of down, you are probably over-training/under-recovering. To avoid over-training and injury, good planning, and deliberate recovery is key.

Bobby Maximus likens the delicate balance of training and recovery to a bank account. The photo on the next page is from one of his seminars A hard training session is -10 points. Minor life stresses are -5 points. A major life stress could be as much as -50. Depending on the severity, it could be even more, knocking you off track for months. Sleeping 8 hours a night is +5 points. Foam rolling is +2 points. Massages are +5 points. Acupuncture is +5. Recovery walks are +1, etc. If at the end of the week your account is in the red, you are setting yourself up for fatigue, injury, and decreased performance.

To keep your account in check, it is essential to get in the habit of prioritizing recovery. This part of fitness is often overlooked and doesn't seem like a big deal until you are injured. If you prioritize recovery BEFORE you become injured, you will save yourself a lot of grief. We will have scheduled de-load weeks in the program (a lighter, lower volume week) and place a LOT of emphasis on self-care between sessions. On the following pages are some of the strategies that Battle Tested encourages implementing to make sure you stay at the top of your game.

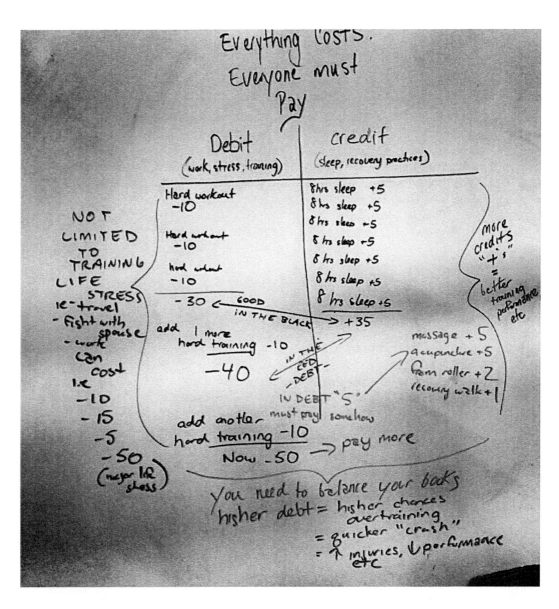

"Everything costs, everyone must pay."

- Bobby Maximus

Sleep A Lot

Your body repairs itself best when you are asleep. If you are consistently not getting enough sleep, your body is again and again not quite able to completely repair tissue damage and replenish energy stores. In an ideal world 8-10 hours a night would be perfect. To most people this sounds impossible. Get as much as you can by rearranging priorities. Is staying up late watching mind-numbing television shows getting you closer to your goals? I didn't think so. I start my day at 4:15am. Quality time alone with my wife usually begins after the kids are in bed. This is a huge struggle for me. It frequently leaves me with very short nights and behind on recovery before my day even gets going. I have to make this up somewhere and mid-day naps seem to be the most convenient way. 8 consecutive hours of sleep would be ideal, but sleep is important wherever you can fit it in.

Drink A Lot of Water

Your body is roughly 60% water. If you're not drinking enough water, what do you suppose is happening to your body? Water clears waste, fuels bodily systems, increases metabolism, and speeds recovery. Research has shown decrease in performance even at 3% water loss. Other studies have shown that even mild dehydration can negatively affect brain function, mood, concentration, and increase anxiety. Chronic dehydration is also a contributor to formation of kidney stones. Most people live in a state of constant dehydration, limiting their capabilities, and slowly their body's ability to recover. 8 glasses (8 ounce) of water a day is a pretty standard recommendation, but for an active person as you will be – you may need more. Honestly, drink enough that your pee is clear. If it is yellow, you probably need more water. Rarely do people have adverse affects of drinking too much water. Hyponatria is actually a very serious medical condition caused by too much water and not enough salts but it's not likely you'll need to worry about it.

Get Bodywork

Most people assume I stress the importance of bodywork because I am a massage therapist, but the opposite is actually true. After years as a strength and conditioning coach, I BECAME a massage therapist because I could no longer deny the importance of bodywork and the benefits it had to offer my athletes. As a competitive volleyball player I could not sleep on my right side for 4 straight years in college. Swedish massage felt good but did little to correct the issue. Occasional physical therapy helped some, but still didn't quite do the trick. Both probably would have made a greater impact on my shoulder health had I done either consistently. Consistency is key. Prevention is much easier than treatment. Equally important is sorting through the available therapists and finding the people and modalities that can help you the most.

Eventually I was referred to a phenomenal massage therapist, Nate Graven, who literally had me feeling the best I had in years after a single session. Within a month of weekly visits, my shoulder felt 100% recovered. This is when I knew that whatever this man was doing was going to change my approach to performance forever. I shadowed him off and on for a year or more, then signed up for massage school.

Good bodywork will improve tissue quality and thus performance by breaking up adhesions and scar tissue, keeping fascia loose and supple, creating space for muscle movement, and improving circulation. Also, it can help restore mechanical advantage by correcting misalignments, lengthening short muscles, and changing the strain on joints. In addition to the benefits to the musculofascial benefits, bodywork can also reduce levels of the stress hormone cortisol, reduce inflammation, increase white blood cells , and increase alertness.

I have had the most relief personally and the most success in my treatment of others with the following therapies: Rolfing or Structural Integration, Myofascial Release, Dry Needling, Active Release, and Positional Release. Looking for therapists who practice any of these modalities is a great place to start. Honestly, the more I learn about bodywork, the less I realize I know and the more modalities I realize there are out there that can have a profound impact on my wellbeing. Experiment with different bodywork styles and different therapists until you find the therapy and the therapists that work best for you.

In addition to occasional visits to Nate, I have an incredible prevention and treatment team in massage therapist Sariah Long and physical therapist Aja Merril. I see them more consistently and they are my immediate treatment plan when something goes wrong. Sariah is a world-class runner who competed in the finals of the 2008 US Olympic Trials for the steeplechase and continues to dominate marathons, ultras, and half marathons now in her early 30s. Aja is a former Division I collegiate volleyball player. This high-level competitive experience makes them perfect for my needs. They understand my mindset and understand the necessity of continuing to perform even while injured. Complete rest is rarely an option. Many post treatment conversations have begun with, "Standard treatment for this would be to rest, ice, avoid these activities, and do these exercises three times a day. Since I know you aren't going to do that, this I need YOU to do…"

Self Myofascial Release

SMR (Self Myofascial Release) is a great form of supplemental massage between visits to a therapist or can be used if working with a therapist is not an option. There are countless tools that can be used for SMR. From something as simple as a foam roller to something as high tech as a Ther-a-gun, there are many options for SMR. Some of our favorite tools are foam rollers, lacrosse balls, T-balls, BT peanuts, bouncy balls, softballs, barbells, and car buffers. The correctives section of this book will go into detail on what these tools are used for and how to use them. Another great resource for self-myofascial release is Dr. Kelly Starrett's book *Becoming a Supple Leopard*.

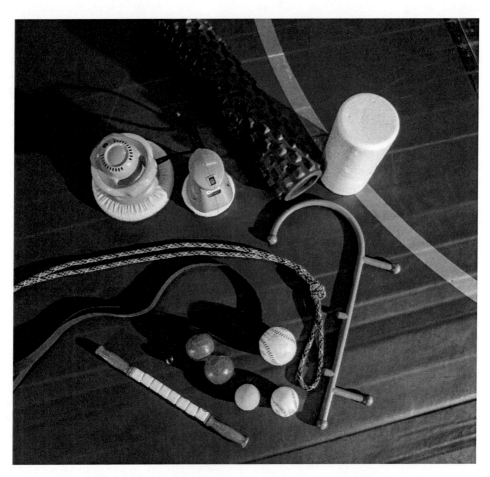

Tools of the trade. These are the recovery tools we use on a daily basis at Competitive Edge.

Ice Baths

One of the most miserable, but rewarding things you can do to speed recovery after a tough workout. Fill a bathtub with several bags of ice and water. Jump in. The first couple of minutes are the worst, but it gets better once you start to go numb. A meta-analysis of 396 research studies on cold-water immersion was published in the Journal of Strength and Conditioning Research in May 2017.

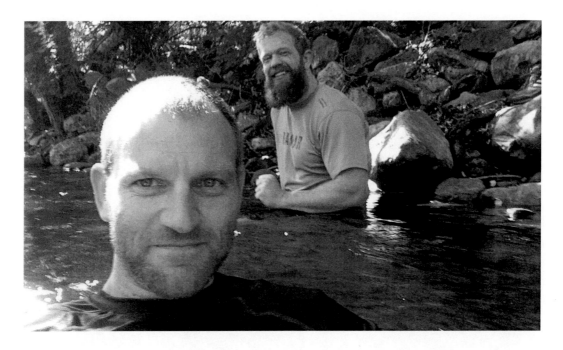

Based on these studies, the recommendation of the analysis was that cold-water immersion for recovery should incorporate two 5-minute immersions at 10 degrees Celsius (50 degrees Fahrenheit) with a 2-minute seated rest between immersions in ambient temperature. I've had great results with a single immersion of 7-10 minutes. Another great variation of this is to sit in very cold rivers or streams like we see Rickson Gracie do in the documentary *Choke*. Due to convection, moving water becomes much colder than standing water, making cold streams an ideal place for icing. There are few things I enjoy more after a long, hard hike than sitting on a rock in the middle of a freezing stream with my feet in the water. This can also be used on a smaller scale. I frequently will fill a small plastic garbage can with ice water to soak my hands and wrists, or to soak my feet and ankles. Ice baths are also a great mental exercise, because for the first 3-4 minutes, they really, really SUCK!

Contrast Bathing
        Similar to ice baths with the difference that it alternates between cold and hot. Start with cold, then after 5-15 minutes move to a warm/hot bath. Continue back and forth 2-3 times. This also works though slightly less effectively in the shower. The shower is more convenient than using a hot tub and a cold tub, therefore I am much more likely to do it. While in the shower post workout, simply alternate between hot water for a few minutes and very cold water for a few minutes.

Ice Massage

I actually really enjoy ice massage. It is a great method for more targeted work. For example, if you are having shoulder, elbow, knee, or ankle pain, this is a fantastic method for direct cold application to the injured joint. I buy re-usable ice cups from www.massagewarehouse.com as shown in the photos below. An alternative is to freeze water in a paper or Styrofoam cup. Once frozen, tear and peel the cup away from top to expose a small portion of ice. Use this to massage inflamed area for 3-4 minutes. Be careful not to go too long to avoid frostbite. 3-4 minutes will be plenty. Smaller areas with less tissue will usually require less time than larger areas (an elbow vs. a shoulder or knee for example). Because of the direct contact of the ice, it isn't necessary to ice for the usual 20 minutes recommended for an ice pack.

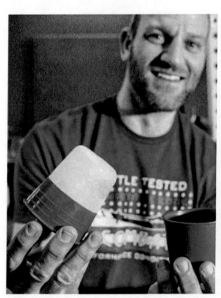 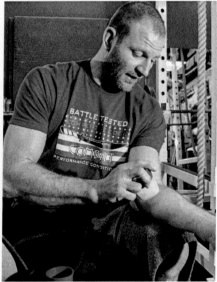

Salt Baths

There is some debate over Epsom salt (magnesium sulfate) baths. They are popularly promoted as a home health remedy, but there seems to be little peer reviewed evidence to the benefits of Epsom salt soaks. The proclaimed benefits of Epsom salt baths are two-fold. One is that they reduce inflammation, which in the case of sprains and other joint injuries, in my experience I agree. The other benefit is supposed to be that your body absorbs magnesium through the skin while soaking in warm/hot water. This is where there is some controversy. An August 2017 article on www.livestrong.com (http://www.livestrong.com) states,

> Despite these claims, there is a lack of peer-reviewed, published research supporting that topical application of magnesium increases body magnesium levels, according to a July 2012 review published in "International Journal of Cosmetic Science." However, skin absorption could occur in the right conditions -- with heat, high salt concentrations or through cut or broken skin -- based on a review article published in the June 2014 issue of "Experimental Biology and Medicine." Additional research is needed to better understand if soaking in Epsom salt leads to any meaningful magnesium absorption through the skin, as well as the health effects of any noted absorption.

One study that does seem to support magnesium absorption is from the School of Biosciences at University of Birmingham, UK. 19 subjects took Epsom salt baths for 7 days, testing blood magnesium levels before and after the baths. Their findings were that the salt baths resulted in higher levels of magnesium, and they concluded Epsom soaks were a safe and easy way to increase magnesium and sulfates in the body.

Whether it is simply placebo, or they truly are beneficial, I find salt baths help me feel better when I am a little run down. At any rate, definitely give it a try and see if you notice a difference. As with the ice bath, you can also use this on a smaller scale for a sprain ankle or sore wrists, etc. For sprains, 2 cups Epsom salt-per-gallon of water is ideal. For baths, I usually put 2-4 cups (depending how much I have on hand) in the tub and fill it with warm water. For recovery, I try not to use hot water, simply because heat won't reduce inflammation. With both ice baths and Epsom salt baths, soaks in general can be beneficial to reduce inflammation. Submersion in water compresses the body, thus helping to push excess fluid back into the lymph system.

Another option if available is a float spa. These are pods with around 1,200 lbs. of Epsom salt that are used for both the benefits of Epsom salt and for sensory deprivation. There is so much salt that you float, weightless and still in the water. In most pods, you can float in darkness or with colored light as well as with or without music. known as sensory deprivation, this is also thought to speed learning as it eliminates distraction. Even The Mind Gym, at SEAL Headquarters in Norfolk, Virginia, is rumored to utilize float tanks to accelerate training. Float spas also seem to show a lot of promise for people suffering

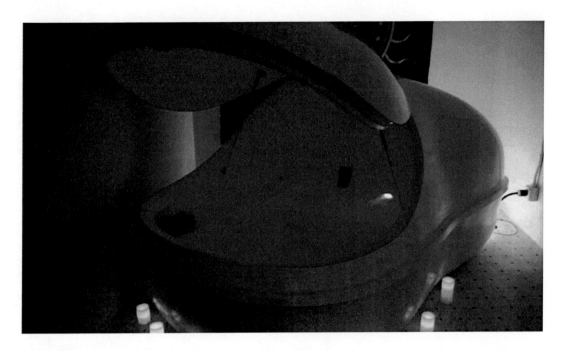

with PTSD, helping with anxiety and lowering cortisol levels among other things. The Laureate Institute for Brain Research in Tulsa, Oklahoma is leading the way in float therapy research, and it will be interesting to see what new things are learned in the coming years.

Get Outside

It is amazing the restorative benefits of spending some time in nature. From previously mentioned soaks in a cold stream, to a leisurely hike or bike ride, to a recreational game your favorite outdoor sport, just about anything outside can be rewarding. Even something strenuous like tire flips, farmer carries, or a Highland Games competition, while challenging, can be oddly therapeutic.

In an article for the journal, Milo Strength, Brian Jones, Ph.D. explains,

The power of nature to reduce stress and anxiety and improve mood has been demonstrated repeatedly. Of the hypotheses explaining this effect, attention restoration theory (ART) is the most widely accepted. ART suggests that natural environments, unlike urban ones, do not induce the type of constant, jarring, mental simulation that leads to cognitive fatigue. Natural environments capture attention in a way that allows for mental relaxation and recovery. People can mentally recover and recharge while in nature. Cognitive fatigue is thought to be a major cause of stress and stress-related conditions, such as anxiety, depression, and insomnia.

Interestingly, performing workouts outside can possibly even improve performance. For several years, I operated a 1,500 square foot man cave called The LAIR, full of rocks, tires, ropes, heavy dumbbells, giant sledge hammers, MMA mats, and a rock climbing cave. It had four big garage doors that we would open up and our workouts would cover every available inch of the garage and parking lot. Something about the fresh air, sunshine, heavy implements, and great training partners guaranteed the workout would be brutal. Without fail, guys would work much harder and push themselves much more than in a regular gym and somehow we always left completely spent yet noticeably refreshed. Workouts at The LAIR quickly became the most psychologically important workouts of my week. I believe training partially outdoors had a lot to do with that.

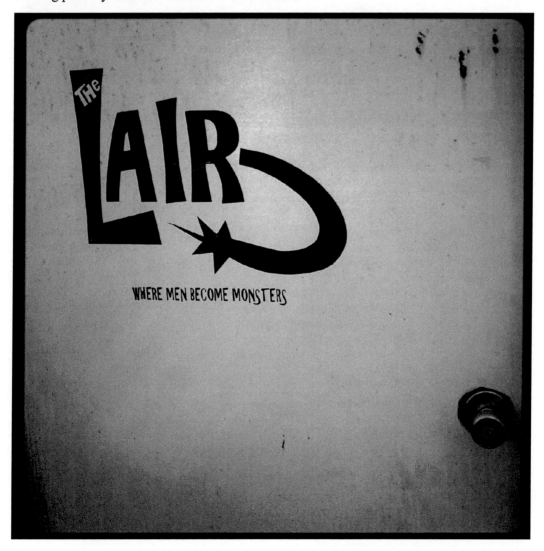

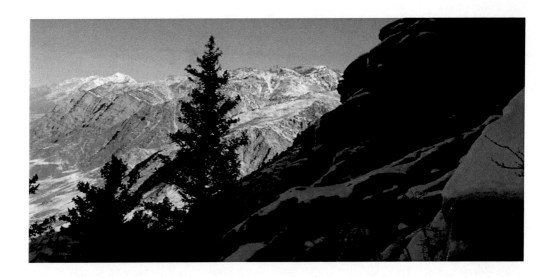

Research to date on "green" fitness has primarily been related to endurance activities, but comparing indoor to outdoor, outdoor exercisers have performed better while maintaining a lower physiological intensity. It makes sense that the same could be true of strength training outside as well. Jones' article in Milo goes on to discuss the performance benefits of time in natural environments. "Reduced stress, improve mood, slower resting heart rate, and lower catabolic hormone levels are all chronic performance enhancers. Optimal fitness adaptation is directly dependent on your recovery capacity."

De-load Workouts

From the programming side, there are also de-load workouts built into the Battle Tested workout plan. Less is often more. While you can expect to work extremely hard through the Battle Tested System, and frequently stumble from the gym, you will also have workouts where you leave feeling great. Don't mistake this for a bad workout. It is impossible to go all out all the time. You will eventually burn out. In addition to the three strength training workouts you do each week, we encourage one day of mobility work. If you opt out of this day, make sure you are getting your foam rolling and mobility work in somewhere throughout the week.

To prevent this, every fourth week is a de-load week. These weeks still include tough workouts, but we quit while there is still some in the tank. You will get a good workout, but not be completely wiped out at the end. Volume is also significantly down. We will often use lower weight than you're capable of, do fewer sets or reps than usual, and work more on single leg and single arm movements. In addition to single limb movements, we will further add to unstable training with band-resisted movements, slosh pipe and water ball workouts, and more targeted agility work. The goal is to challenge our bodies in different ways than the previous three weeks without lifting as much weight and without beating ourselves up too much. -111.919206

PART II
Making it Personal

"Find your weaknesses, make friends with them, then beat them to death."
- Chris Spealler

We all have different needs. We have different goals. Different things motivate and inspire us. Different things can hold us back. If I just hand you a program to follow without considering these things, you might make progress. You might gain strength. You might increase your durability. Or you may fail miserably because our plan didn't line up with your reality. The following chapters are designed to improve your capability to succeed. They contain ideas to remain disciplined and focused on your goals as well as the opportunity to take an in-depth look at your body and correct any weak links that might be holding you back. In strength and conditioning, not addressing a weakness increases our potential for injury as we try to progress. We assess pain, posture and movement and provide you detailed instructions for addressing issues you might be facing. These corrective protocols can become part of your pre-workout warm-up, can be done on post workout, or performed on days off as active recovery.

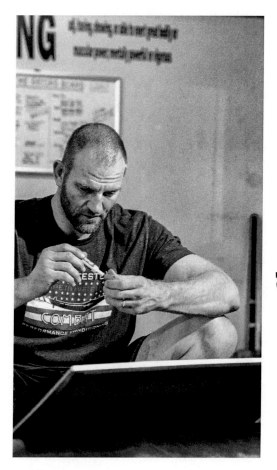

Chapter 5
Designing Your Program

Chapter 5 – Designing Your Program

Start with a Goal

You have to know where you are going if you ever intend to get there. Someone can still become very fit without a clear goal, but it is comparable to starting out on a road trip without a destination just to enjoy the ride. I'm all about enjoying the journey, but as soldiers, fighters, climbers, or athletes of any kind, there must always be a goal. Lack of solid goals gives birth to complacency and laziness. Not having a goal means you cannot have a "why". You WILL NOT work as hard, or make as much progress if you don't have a pre-planned destination. Without a "why", you will eventually stop, content with where you are. Many of you may know what your goal is. Do you have a vague goal, or a specific goal? It is easy to say, "I want to be a better fighter," or "I want to be stronger." How do you quantify that? How do you know when you get there? What are the specifics that detail your goal?

Set S.M.A.R.T Goals

A common strategy for effective goal setting is to use the acronym SMART. Here's how it works. A good goal must be:

S	=	**Specific**
M	=	**Measurable**
A	=	**Attainable**
R	=	**Relevant**
T	=	**Time Bound**

Specific - What exactly do you want to do, and why do you want to do it? What and who will it involve to make it happen?

Measurable - Goals have to be measurable to work. You need an endpoint to know when the goal has been achieved. This also helps to plan the steps you need to take along the way.

Attainable - Is your goal something you can achieve? Is it realistic? Does this goal dependent solely on your efforts, or is their someone else who has power over your success?

Relevant - Make sure you have a why. Does this goal align with your other goals, or are you chasing rabbits?

Time Bound - A good goal needs to have a dead-line. Without a deadline, there is no urgency, and it is easy to procrastinate and put off putting forth the effort required to reach your goal.

Determine Your Starting Point

Once you know what your goal is, you need to determine where you are starting. You know where you're going, but where are you coming from? How close are you to your goal? What limitations do you have that will keep you from meeting your goal? What obstacles might you encounter along the way? Obstacles and limitations can be physical, mental, or emotional. They can be personal, or determined by someone or something completely outside of your control. The first step is to assess where you are currently at. Once you know that, it is only a matter of determining the most effective way from point A to point. The next chapter will take you through a physical assessment prior to beginning the Battle Tested program.

Working Backwards From Your Goal

It is important to work backwards from your goal. Life and fitness are both progressive and many target goals move and change constantly. When I finally reach my black belt in Jiu-Jitsu, do I stop there? Of course not. If I add 50 lbs. to my max dead-lift, will I be content enough to stop trying to improve? I hope not. Goals can be huge. But reaching big, big goals is a process of meeting one smaller goal after another. You are much more likely to reach your ultimate goal by breaking it into smaller, more manageable portions. I didn't decide, "I'm going to get a black belt in Jiu-Jitsu someday," without understanding there are other belts along the way. The ultimate goal can be hugely time consuming, marked by smaller successes along the way. If my strength goal is to hex bar dead-lift three times my bodyweight this year, where do I have to be three months from now? Where do I have to be 6 months from now? This gets tricky because I know I will make slower and slower progress the closer I get to my goal, but without a plan in place, I don't stand a chance.

Sometimes, the end goal is simply survival. And it must be broken down into tiny, tiny bits that are all you can handle at any given time. While speaking about the events in the movie Lone Survivor, Marcus Luttrell talked about being alone, with a broken back, paralyzed from the waist down. He explained that he took a rock, reached out, and drew a line in the dirt. He told himself, "I'm going to crawl until my feet hit that line, and if I'm still alive, I'm going to do it again." Marcus crawled that way for seven miles.

What are your goals? What are the necessary steps to reach it? How willing are you to dig in and do whatever it takes to reach it?

Dominate Your Goals

Nearly everyone has goals, whether fitness or otherwise. Most people also decide to make the change. Where most people struggle is actually following through and doing the things that need to be done to make the change. It is easy to pursue a goal when motivated. But motivation comes and goes. The key is not to rely on motivation, rather to have the discipline to relentlessly chase your goals NO MATTER WHAT. Here are several ideas to keep you on track.

Read Bible 15-20
minutes 1st thing daily
✓ JOHN
MARK
PSALMS

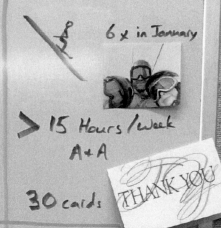

6 x in January

> 15 Hours/week
A+A

30 cards

THANK YOU

Finish Bathroom
Remodels

12 new
Police Officers

┌─────────────────┐
│ Schedule/Plan   │
│ BATTLE TESTED   │
│ Seminar   │
└─────────────────┘

Get Published
in Men's Health
Magazine!

Pain Free Hips/low
Back

3 naps/week

Plank @ 100 lbs.
> 4:47
Plank @ 200 lbs.
> 3:08

TGU
> 28,000 kg
in 24 hours

Hex Bar Dead-lift

3.2x Bodyweight

Vision Boards

      Vision boards are awesome. The idea behind a vision board is to spend time each day visually acknowledging your goal. Whether you use a white board, poster board, sticky notes, or window markers, write down or post a picture of your goals on the board. You can have a single goal, or separate your board into 2, 4, or 6 different goals. I like to use a 6 space board with a goal for each of the following categories:

1) God, 2) Family/Friends, 3) Projects, 4) Business, 5) Health, and 6) Performance Goals

      Most goals should be fairly attainable, shorter term goals such as lose 5-10 lbs., send out 30 thank you cards, read 4 books, improve your squat by 20 lbs., etc. Long term general goals like "be a better father" are great, but use your vision board for specific stepping stones toward that primary goal. On the top right corner of my board on the previous page, is my family square. Steps toward being a better husband and father are to ski with my kids at least six times during the month (a photo helps make it more real) and to spend at least 15 hours of quality time alone with my wife each week. Other visual cues are the thank you card, the stick figure skier, and the Guinness World Records logo.

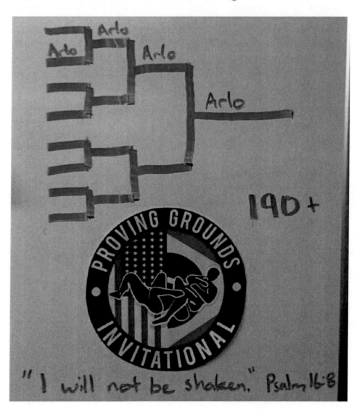

On the previous page is another portion of a past vision board when I was preparing for a specific event. I put this on my vision board months before I was even invited to the tournament. I included the weight division I planned on competing in, then mapped out what the bracket would look like if I won (remember, we are always in it for first), and focused on that. I put the tournament logo, because it was a visual representation of my primary goal - participating in the tournament. I knew as a purple belt who hadn't competed consistently in several years I would go into the tournament as a major underdog. As an underdog, "I will not be shaken," became my mantra. The complete verse, Proverbs 16:8 says, "I have set the Lord always before me. Because He is at my right hand, I will not be shaken." I screen printed Psalm 16:8 on my fight shorts as a constant visual reminder I could look down at any time. I ended up competing in the 160-190 division and losing a high-paced first match to accomplished brown belt Isiah Wright, but I walked onto the mat more mentally prepared than I have ever been.

Once you have created your board, place it where you will see it immediately when you wake up. Each morning, look at your board for 3 minutes as soon as you wake up and focus on what needs to be done to achieve each goal. This starts your day out on the right track, reminding you what you should make a priority for the day. Each night, right before bed, focus on your board again for 3 minutes. Doing this, it's not unusual to even dream about your goals and how to reach them. There are mornings I wake up motivated to dominate my goals before I even look at the board.

Once you have committed to focusing your mind on your goals a mere 6 minutes a day, the next step is to relentlessly pursue these short term goals until you meet them. It should be a competition, or game of sorts, to see how fast you can check things off and put up another goal that will get you closer to long-term success. Put up a vision board immediately. It doesn't have to be perfect, so don't put it off. Put it where you will see it first thing in the morning and right before bed. Commit to using it consistently. Then, chase your dreams.

IMMEDIATE ACTION #5
Vision Board

Start your vision board NOW! Use the categories I listed, or make your own. Regardless if you plan to use a vision board or not, fill in the board on the following page now for practice and take a picture of it with your phone. This way, you can reflect on it anytime, anywhere. If you choose to make a bigger, easier seen vision board at home or at work, take a picture of that board when it is done. If you really want to commit, share the photo of your board online with the Battle Tested Tribe and let us help keep you accountable.

Eliminate Distractions

Distractions are everywhere. There is a common thought that it takes roughly 10,000 hours to become an expert at something (Malcolm Gladwell suggests this time may vary, but you get the point). Looking at your goals, you know where you need to spend your time. Time is a huge obstacle for people successfully achieving their goals. There are obviously things unrelated to our goals that need to be addressed. Time with family is priority. Work is essential. Sleep is necessary. But, what about all of those other things? Following the 10,000 hour idea, I am much closer to being an expert on social media than I care to admit. How much time per day do you spend browsing Facebook? How many hours a week do you watch Netflix? Are either of these things getting you closer to your goals, or are they sucking away valuable time that could be dedicated to your resolutions? What things can you cut back on or cut out completely that are distracting you from the things you should be doing? You are rarely stagnant in pursuit of your goals. You are always getting closer to them or further away from them. The less time you spend distracted by unnecessary things in your life, the more time you can spend on the things you decide matter.

Train With Intent

It is easy to go to the gym and go through the motions. Easy to know what the goal is, but go to the gym without a plan and do whatever sounds fun for the day. Lacking structure, lacking a game plan, lacking intent will keep you from reaching your goals.

My fitness goals are always performance based. About a year ago, I came to the realization that I often just go through the motions. I work hard in the gym, and I train often, but I realized I often lack intent. I have goals, but don't always spend time thinking about them before a workout or before Jiu-Jitsu class. I love Jiu-Jitsu, but that sometimes gets in the way of my goals. I actually draw a lot of joy just going through the motions. Win or lose, I spar and I have FUN! Jiu-Jitsu is a good workout, great stress relief, and quality time I can spend with friends. Too often I can get beat soundly and leave class content and smiling. Other days I beat up on a bunch of newer guys and leave smiling. Is it bad to enjoy every day? Not necessarily. What is bad is that I still often go to class unfocused when I know if I spend a few minutes reviewing my goals, and focusing specifically on what I know I need to work on, I not only grapple better, but I get much more out of my training session. It takes Jiu-Jitsu from just another fun day at class to actually making progress toward my grappling goals. Training complacently doesn't get me closer to my goals. Training with intent does.

So how do you train with intent? Your new vision board can help. If you train in the morning your goals should be fresh in your mind. If you train mid-day or evening, another 3 minutes looking at your vision board can make a world of difference. If you took a picture of your vision board with your phone, you can always have it at your fingertips. If not your vision board, just dedicate a few minutes prior to training to reflect on your goals. Spend some time before, or even as you warm up for a workout, mentally reviewing your goals and what you need to achieve for the day to progress toward them. Remind yourself before every workout why you are there and you are much more likely to work hard and stay motivated.

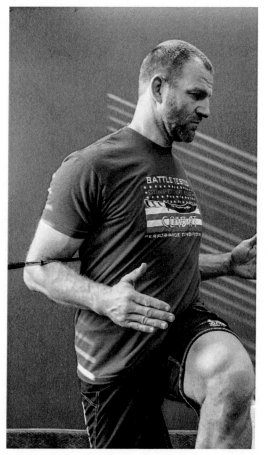

Chapter 6
Self Assessment

Chapter 6 - Self Assessment

The assessment process can be extremely complicated, or it can be fairly simple. There are hundreds of potential function tests that can be done to identify any limitations. If you want to go that route, an experienced physical therapist can help you with that. For the purpose of this book, we will briefly assess pain, posture, and movement. Exploring these three areas will serve to direct our training efforts. If you are experiencing issues outside of this basic assessment, you should seek the help of a qualified professional.

1) Pain

The first thing we will take into consideration is pain. In physical therapist Gray Cook's popular Functional Movement Screen, seven different movements are scored on a scale of 0-3. If there any pain caused by any movement, that movement scores a 0, regardless of how well it is performed. If you have pain, something is wrong. When we begin training, eliminating this pain should be a top priority.

Do you have pain? Headaches, joint pain, muscle pain, can all give us clues as to what our corrective focus needs to be. Assessing pain is quite simple. What hurts? Why? Many things can cause pain, and it is far outside the scope of this book and my expertise to diagnose any medical conditions. However, there are certainly patterns that show themselves again and again in those I work with and they are worth considering when you are evaluating yourself. Often, where we have pain, will guide us in the things to look for during posture and movement. Remember the mobility vs. stability chart from Chapter 2? If a joint hurts, it could be because it isn't stable or mobile enough. Not only that, it could be because the joint above or below it isn't stable or mobile enough. Here are some common pain patterns I see on a daily basis:

Headaches - frequently due to dehydration or overly tight neck muscles

Neck Pain/Shoulder Pain/Upper Back Pain - frequently caused by tight internal shoulder rotators and weak external rotators as well as head forward posture

Lower Back Pain - frequently caused by tight hip flexors and weak/inactive hip extensors and core muscles and/or poor hip mobility

Knee Pain - frequently caused by tight quadriceps muscles, weak hamstring muscles, and/or poor hip or ankle mobility

Heel Pain - frequently caused by tight calves and plantar fascia and/or poor ankle mobility

In addition to these pain patterns, there are also different identifying factors that can help us determine what the source of our pain might be. Here are some basic guidelines that can help identify what we might be dealing with.

Soft tissue - Pain throughout range of motion

Tendonitis - Pain only with active range of motion

Bursitis - Pain with active or passive range of motion

Nerve - Numbness and tingling, possible loss of strength

2) Posture   As previously discussed, the places we are experiencing pain can guide our postural assessment. If we are experiencing pain somewhere, we know to examine both the place of the pain and what is happening at the joint above and the joint below the pain. Posture serves as a good tool to help determine what is causing the pain. When we see deviation from neutral posture, something is tight, and something is weak. Sometimes these deviations result in a pain pattern, and sometimes they do not. However, if we have pain, we can frequently identify a possible cause through postural assessment. If we do not have pain, a postural assessment can preemptively warn us of something that may become a problem, so that we can begin to address it. Even in the absence of pain, poor posture can lead to mobility restrictions and decreased performance potential.

Posture can be affected by many factors, but most commonly, by what we do the most of. People who sit at desks all day frequently have rounded forward shoulders, and pelvic tilt. Some very athletic people, who sit on a bike a lot, will likely have similar issues. One of the first questions I ask clients with severe postural issues is, "What do you do for work?" Eight hours a day in any position is going to start to change the body. Fighters also frequently have poor posture. Boxers are taught to keep their chin down and shoulders forward while jiu-jitsu guys keep their chin tucked and back rounded to roll easier. It doesn't have to be career related either. People who are taller than the majority of those they are surrounded by, will also likely have rounded forward shoulders, head forward posture and their head tilted down. When you are taller than everyone, you are always looking down, and your body adapts.

On the following pages, we will look at some anterior, lateral, and posterior drawings of the human body, then evaluate some actual photographs of veteran and former collegiate rugby player, Jake. We had him fake some issues, so he's not as screwed up as he appears in some of these pictures. Get with your battle buddy and do a postural assessment together. Use the drawings and cues as a checklist for your own posture.

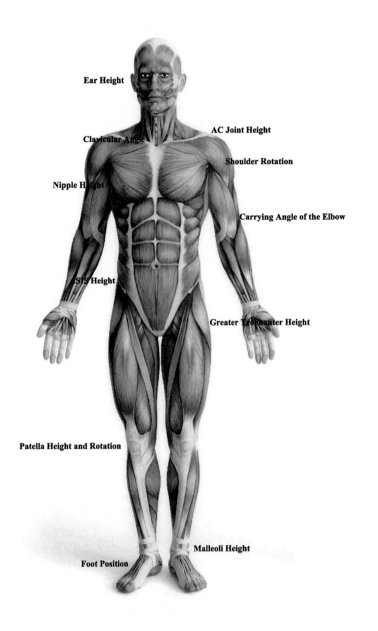

Ear Height

AC Joint Height

Clavicular Angle

Shoulder Rotation

Nipple Height

Carrying Angle of the Elbow

ASIS Height

Greater Trochanter Height

Patella Height and Rotation

Malleoli Height

Foot Position

Anterior View

*Straight vertical line from nose to chin to sternum to navel to pubis symphysis

*Eye height should be even bilaterally; head tilt

*Ear height should be even bilaterally; head tilt

*Clavicles should have the same angle (6-20 degrees upslope from medial to lateral)

*AC (acromioclavicular) joint height should be even bilaterally

*Nipple height should be even bilaterally

*Elbow height should be even bilaterally

*Carrying angle (bend of the elbow when palms forward) should be even bilaterally

*ASIS (anterior superior iliac spine) should be even

      Pelvic tilt

      Pelvic rotation

*Greater trochanters should be even bilaterally

*Patella height should be even bilaterally

*Patella should be line up above 1st and second toe

      Internal or external rotation of the knee

      Genu valgum or genu varom (knees caving in, or bowing out)

*Medial malleoli should be slightly higher than lateral malleoli, but even bilaterally

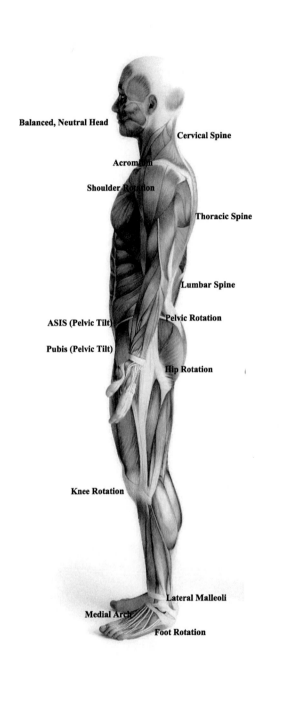

Balanced, Neutral Head

Cervical Spine

Acromion

Shoulder Rotation

Thoracic Spine

Lumbar Spine

ASIS (Pelvic Tilt)

Pelvic Rotation

Pubis (Pelvic Tilt)

Hip Rotation

Knee Rotation

Lateral Malleoli

Medial Arch

Foot Rotation

Lateral View

*Straight vertical line from earlobe to acromium process to elbow to greater trochanter to

center of knee joint to slightly anterior to the lateral malleoli

*Head position balanced over thorax, not pushed forward

*Normal lordotic curve in cervical spine

*No internal rotation of the shoulders

*Normal kyphotic curve in thoracic spine

*Normal lordotic curve in lumbar spine

*ASIS of pelvis should be in line with pubis; no anterior or posterior pelvic tilt

*No right or left rotation of the pelvis

*No external or internal hip rotation

*No external or internal rotation of the knees

*No external or internal rotation of the feet

*Normal medial arch of the feet

Ear Height

Base of Skull Height

Trapezius Symmetry

Acromium Height

Medial Angle of Scapula
Rotation and Distance from Spine

Inferior Angle of Scapula Height

Iliac Crest Height

PSIS Height

Gluteal Crease Height

Popliteal Fossa Height

Gastrocnemius

Achilles Tendon

Calcaneus

Posterior View

*Straight vertical line through spine from occiput to coccyx

*Ear height even bilaterally; head tilt

*Base of skull height even bilaterally; head tilt

*No cervical rotation

*Trapezius symmetry bilaterally

*Acromium height even bilaterally

*Medial angle of scapula equal distance from spine; no abduction or adduction

*Inferior angle of scapula height even bilaterally; no elevation or depression

*Scapular rotation even bilaterally

*Iliac crest height even bilaterally

*PSIS (posterior superior iliac spine) height even bilaterally

*Gluteal crease height even bilaterally

*Popliteal fossa height even bilaterally

*Medial malleoli should be slightly higher than lateral malleoli, but even bilaterally

*Straight vertical line through gastrocnemius, achilles tendon, and calcaneus

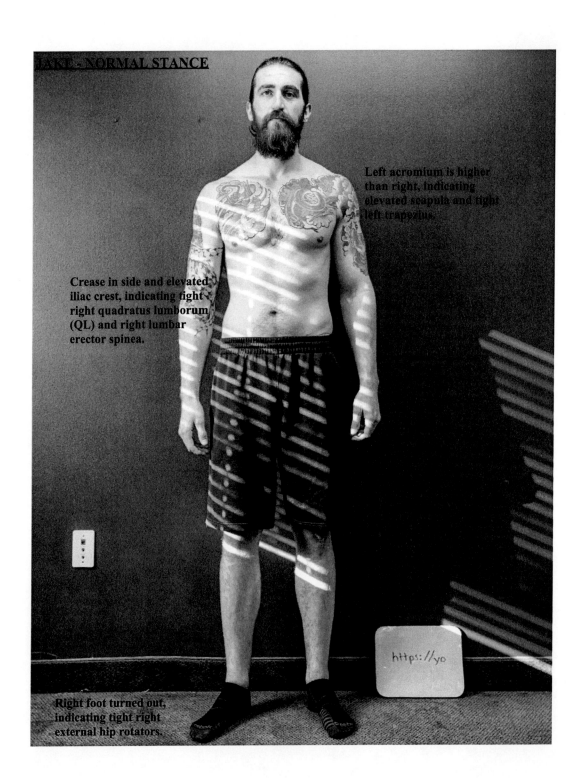

JAKE - NORMAL STANCE

Left acromium is higher than right, indicating elevated scapula and tight left trapezius.

Crease in side and elevated iliac crest, indicating tight right quadratus lumborum (QL) and right lumbar erector spinea.

Right foot turned out, indicating tight right external hip rotators.

https://yo

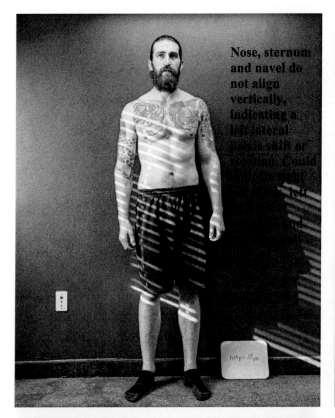

Nose, sternum and navel do not align vertically, indicating a left lateral pelvis shift or rotation. Could indicate right [...] left [...] and [...]

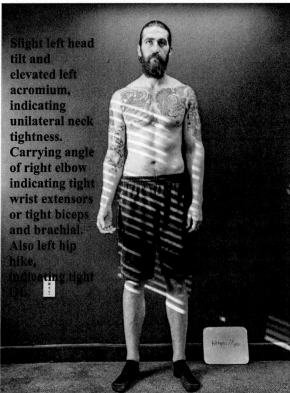

Slight left head tilt and elevated left acromium, indicating unilateral neck tightness. Carrying angle of right elbow indicating tight wrist extensors or tight biceps and brachial. Also left hip hike, indicating tight QL.

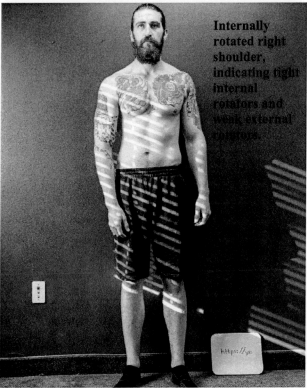

Internally rotated right shoulder, indicating tight internal rotators and weak external rotators.

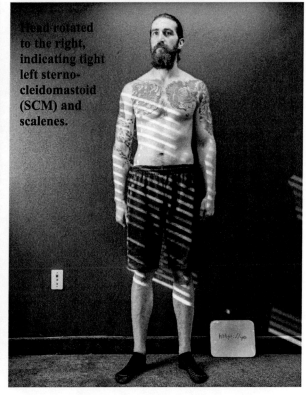

Head rotated to the right, indicating tight left sterno-cleidomastoid (SCM) and scalenes.

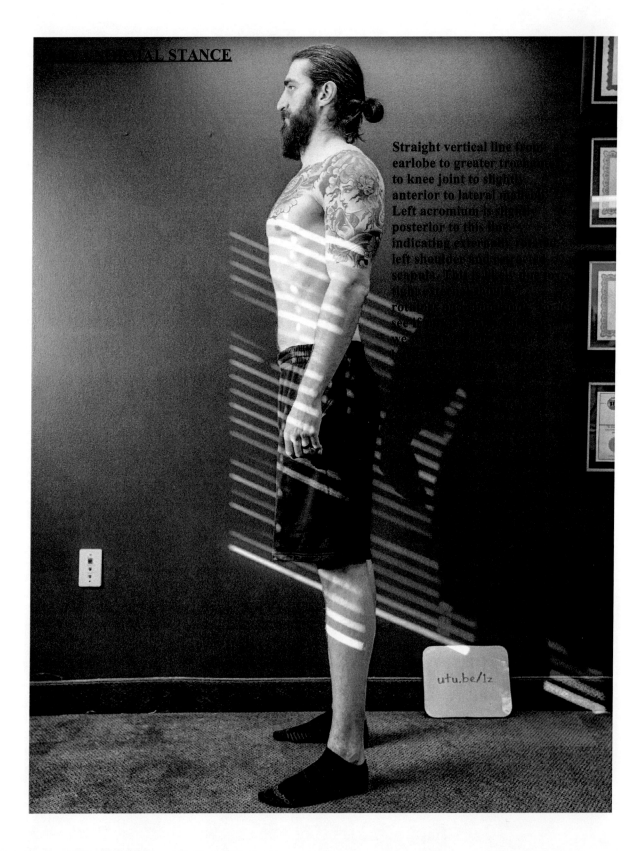

NORMAL STANCE

Straight vertical line from earlobe to greater trochanter to knee joint to slightly anterior to lateral malleolus. Left acromium is slightly posterior to this line, indicating externally rotated left shoulder and protracted scapula. This indicates tight pectorals and internally rotated arm/shoulder. Let's see if we can fix some of these issues.

utu.be/1z

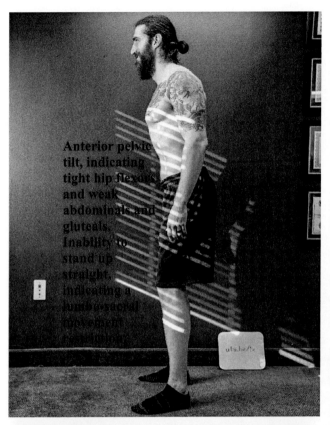

Anterior pelvic tilt, indicating tight hip flexors and weak abdominals and gluteals. Inability to stand up straight, indicating a lumbo-sacral movement resolution.

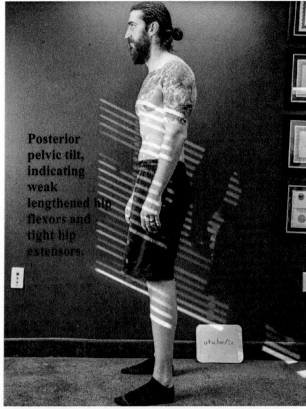

Posterior pelvic tilt, indicating weak lengthened hip flexors and tight hip extensors.

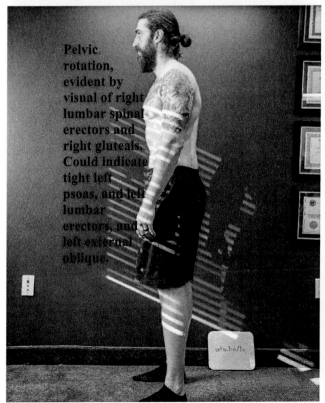

Pelvic rotation, evident by visual of right lumbar spinal erectors and right gluteals. Could indicate tight left psoas, and left lumbar erectors, and left external oblique.

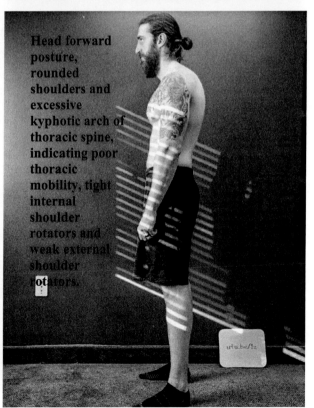

Head forward posture, rounded shoulders and excessive kyphotic arch of thoracic spine, indicating poor thoracic mobility, tight internal shoulder rotators and weak external shoulder rotators.

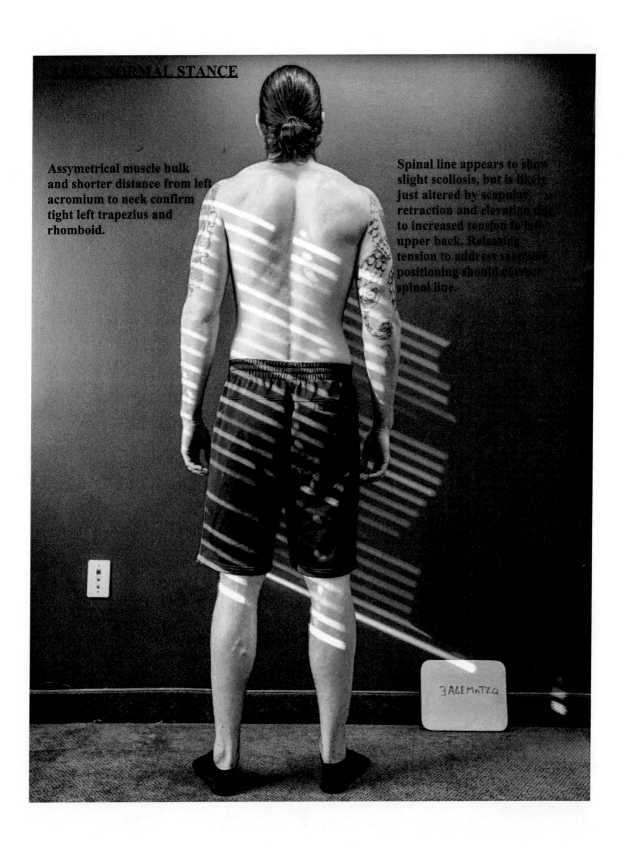

JAKE: NORMAL STANCE

Assymetrical muscle bulk
and shorter distance from left
acromium to neck confirm
tight left trapezius and
rhomboid.

Spinal line appears to show
slight scoliosis, but is likely
just altered by scapular
retraction and elevation due
to increased tension in left
upper back. Releasing
tension to address scapular
positioning should correct
spinal line.

3ALEMnTZQ

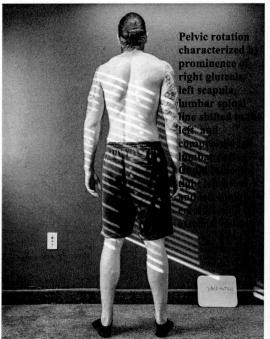

Pelvic rotation characterized by prominence of right gluteals, left scapula, lumbar spinal line shifted to the left, and compressed lumbar [...] right [...] and [...]

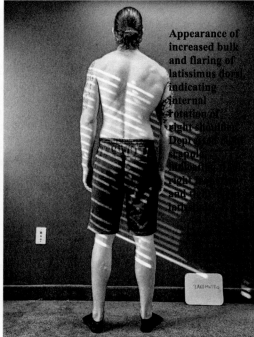

Appearance of increased bulk and flaring of latissimus dorsi, indicating internal rotation of right shoulder. Depressed right scapula [...] right [...] and [...]

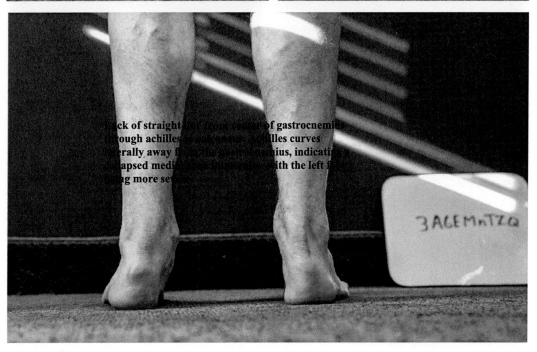

Lack of straight line from center of gastrocnemius through achilles to calcaneus. Achilles curves laterally away from the gastrocnemius, indicating collapsed medial arch bilaterally, with the left foot being more severe.

3) Movement

Once we examine static posture, then we need to see how posture changes once the body starts to move. We need to assess joint range of motion and the ability of the joints to maintain strength and stability through this range of motion. There are a few very natural movements people should be able to do, that we often lose the capability to do as we go through life. They can be limited by injury, imbalances, or just the loss of mobility and stability to perform the movements simply because we stop doing them.

The Deep Squat

Hour after hour, we sit behind desks, steering wheels, and dinner tables, getting weaker, decreasingly mobile, and less pleasing to the eyes. Our posture suffers, our core gets lazy, our backs weaken, our hip flexors grow tighter, and we spend half our gym time trying to figure out why everything hurts.

Contrarily, across the third world, people drop effortlessly into rock bottom squats and sit there as long as necessary. Old ladies can sit in a deep squat preparing food and cooking for hours. Their balance is solid, their range of motion unrestricted, and unsurprisingly, they have less incidence of low back pain. Chairs are few, toilets don't exist, and if anyone owns a bike, it comes with at least two passengers.

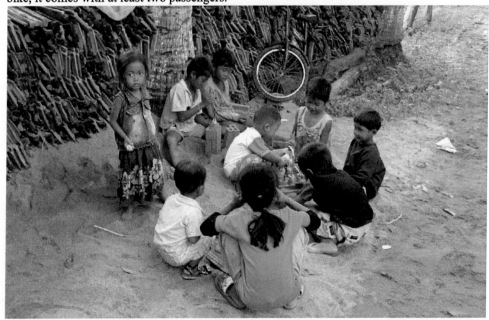

Children can easily sit in a deep squat playing for hours without ever being taught how to do it. In many countries, this ability carries on throughout the remainder of their lives. In the United States, as we grow older, we unwittingly figure out a way to screw it all up.

100

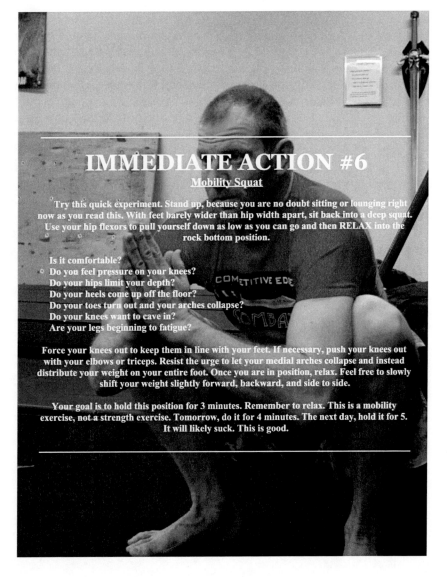

IMMEDIATE ACTION #6
Mobility Squat

Try this quick experiment. Stand up, because you are no doubt sitting or lounging right now as you read this. With feet barely wider than hip width apart, sit back into a deep squat. Use your hip flexors to pull yourself down as low as you can go and then RELAX into the rock bottom position.

Is it comfortable?
Do you feel pressure on your knees?
Do your hips limit your depth?
Do your heels come up off the floor?
Do your toes turn out and your arches collapse?
Do your knees want to cave in?
Are your legs beginning to fatigue?

Force your knees out to keep them in line with your feet. If necessary, push your knees out with your elbows or triceps. Resist the urge to let your medial arches collapse and instead distribute your weight on your entire foot. Once you are in position, relax. Feel free to slowly shift your weight slightly forward, backward, and side to side.

Your goal is to hold this position for 3 minutes. Remember to relax. This is a mobility exercise, not a strength exercise. Tomorrow, do it for 4 minutes. The next day, hold it for 5. It will likely suck. This is good.

How was it? Want to make your daily deep squat more interesting and increasingly beneficial? Focusing on your goals is difficult. Focusing on them with distractions is even harder. Focusing while experiencing pain and discomfort can be nearly impossible, but that is exactly what you will be training yourself to do. People usually give up on their goals either when the distractions are too great or the process is too uncomfortable. This daily mobility drill is also a great time to focus on your goals. Remember your vision board? Next time you look at your vision board for 3 minutes, do it while holding the deep squat. If you have a single primary goal, focus on that. Focus on what you need to accomplish today to reach your goal. If you are about to workout, spend some time thinking about why you are about to do the workout you are about to do. Get your mind focused on and primed for a productive training session. Maybe your goal is a martial arts promotion, an upcoming tournament, or an MMA fight. If you are a fighter with a fight coming up, focus on your opponent. Visualize what he does and how you will outwork and outperform him. Win the fight in your mind long before you ever step in the cage.

Dedicate this daily time to your goal. WHY do you want to achieve this goal and what are you willing to sacrifice to get there. Spending a few minutes each day focusing intently on your goal will make a tremendous impact on whether or not your reach it. Improving your hip mobility and core stability while you focus on your goal makes this quick drill one of the most productive ways you can start your day.

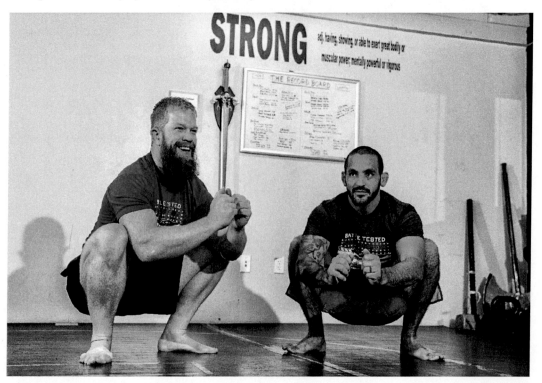

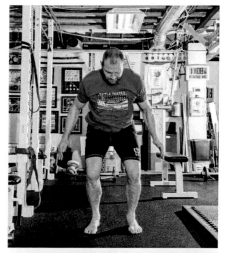

The Squat Jump

In addition to seeing if you can lower into a deep squat or not, we want to look at what happens when you jump. The faster a movement, the more load is placed on the joints and the greater the demand for stability.

Can you load for a jump and then execute a jump without your knees collapsing in or bowing out? Upon landing, how well do you absorb the landing through flexing the hips, knees and, ankles? Do you land hard, or soft? Do your knees cave in on landing?

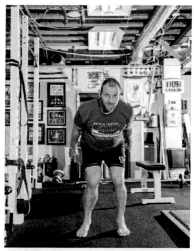

Because females have wider hips, resulting in a greater Q angle (the angle at which the femur meets the tibia), they are more likely to cave at the knees during takeoff and landing, and are at greater risk for knee pain and injury. That being said, it can happen to males as well and happens particularly in people with weak or inactive gluteals.

If you observe knee caving during the jump in yourself or your battle buddy, being aware of it is the first and most important step to preventing it. Just realizing it is happening and focusing on avoiding it can go a long way. The stabilization portion of the Battle Tested workout program is focused on fixing these issues.

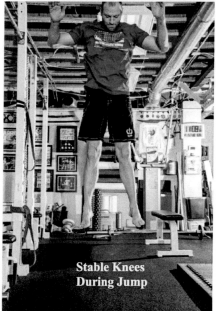

Stable Knees During Jump

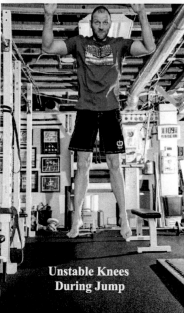

Unstable Knees During Jump

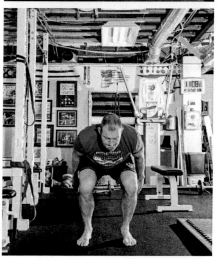

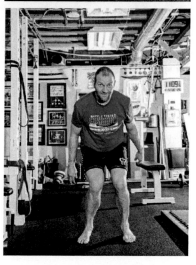

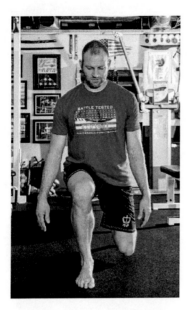

Good knee alignment during lunge.

The Lunge

Like the squat, the lunge is also a great assessment for knee stability. During the lunge however, we reduce the base of support, making any stability issues more pronounced.

The lunge should be performed with an upright torso, and the front heel flat on the ground. Assess the lunge both from the front and from the side, looking for balance and stability issues, ability to hold upright posture during the movement, and technical proficiency.

If you do poorly on the lunge test, being aware of where your technique is breaking down and attempting to correct it goes a long way toward correcting the problems. In addition, you may benefit from the exercises in Corrective Protocols 1 and 2. If your front heel is coming off the floor, focus on Foam Roll Calf, the Gravity Drop, and the Tennis Ball Squat. If you are having trouble with knee alignment, focus on the Dead Bug, Stability Ball Hip Thrust and the 1-leg Hip Extension.

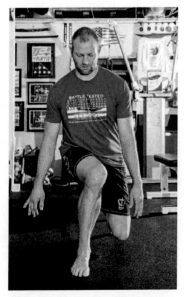

Poor knee alignment during lunge.

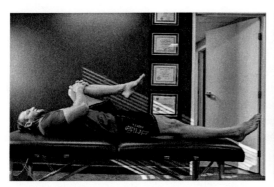 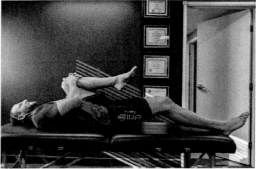

Normal result for Thomas Test, when left knee is pulled toward chest, right leg remains flat on table.   *Poor result for Thomas Test, when left knee is pulled toward chest, the right leg elevates off the table.*

The Thomas Test

The Thomas Test is a test to assess hip flexion contracture. Contracture is essentially a shortening of the muscles and fascia that prevents the hip joint from returning to a neutral position. Often the connective tissue becomes fibrous, restricting and limiting normal movement.

For the Thomas Test, lie supine on a therapy table or on the floor and pull one knee toward your chest, while attempting to keep the opposite knee flat on the table. If the straight leg elevates when the opposite knee is pulled toward the chest, the test is positive for hip flexion contracture. In contracture, the tissue should feel tight and unhealthy as well. If the tissue is instead soft, there is likely another issue such as a joint capsule tightness.

If you do poorly on the Thomas Test, you would benefit from doing the exercises in Corrective Protocol 2. Focus on the Peanut Roll and the Barbell Roll for the quadriceps, the Lacrosse Ball Psoas Release, the Hip Flexor Progressions, and the PNF Quadriceps Stretch.

Ely's Test

For the Ely Test, lie prone on a therapy table, or on the floor. Prior to knee flexion, the hip should lay flat on the table. If you are doing the assessment with your battle buddy, have them passively flex (bend) one knee and watch what happens to the hips. If the hip on the same side as the flexed knee also flexes, lifting the hip off of the table, the test is positive for tight rectus femoris (the most superficial quad muscle that attaches on the ASIS of the pelvis, crosses the hip joint and the knee joint and inserts at the tibial tuberosity). If doing the test alone, actively flex the knee and note what happens at the hip.

If you do poorly on Ely's Test, you would benefit from incorporating the exercises in Corrective Protocol 2. Focus on the Peanut Roll and the Barbell Roll for the quadriceps, the Hip Flexor Progressions, and the PNF Quadriceps stretch.

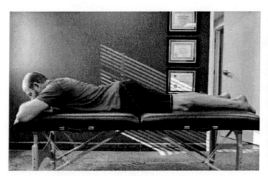

Beginning position for Ely Test.

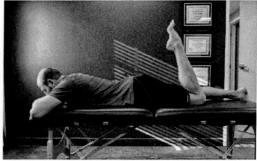

Normal result for Ely Test, the knee bends without elevation of the hips.

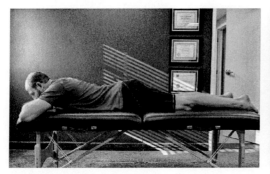

Beginning position for Ely Test.

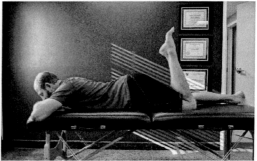

Poor result for Ely Test, the hip elevates off the table and the lordotic arch of the lumbar spine increases when the knee bends.

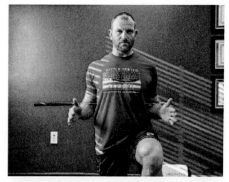

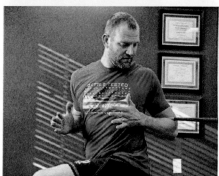

Golf Club Rotation

The golf club rotation is used to assess thoracic rotation. Begin in half kneeling position (like a lunge, but with the back knee firmly on the ground), with a golf club behind your back held by the bends of your elbows. Keep the club flat against your back and rotate as far as possible over the front leg. Only rotate as far as you can before one side of the club comes off of the back. Doing this is a half kneeling position limits lumbar rotation requiring more movement from from thoracic spine.

If you have trouble with this movement, you can continue to use this stretch to improve the movement, as well as incorporating the correctives in Corrective Protocol 3. Focus on the Foam Roll and Peanut Roll for the Upper Back, PVC Mobility, PNF Shoulders, and the Band Pull-apart

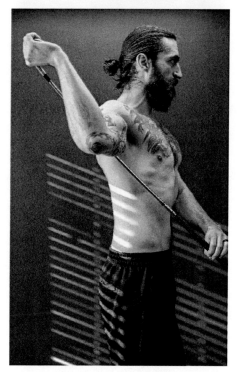

Golf Club Shoulder Rotation

The golf club shoulder rotation is used to assess external rotation of the shoulder. Ideally, with shoulder abducted to 90 degrees (elbow at shoulder height), you will be able to externally rotate until your forearm is in line with your torso or beyond. If you are lacking this ability to externally rotate your shoulder, you can use this stretch to improve it and also can incorporate the correctives in Corrective Protocol 3. Focus on the MB Chest, PVC Mobility, PNF Shoulders, Scapular Wall Slides, and the Abducted Shoulder External Rotation.

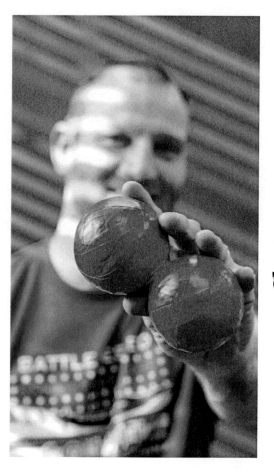

Chapter 7
Corrective Protocols

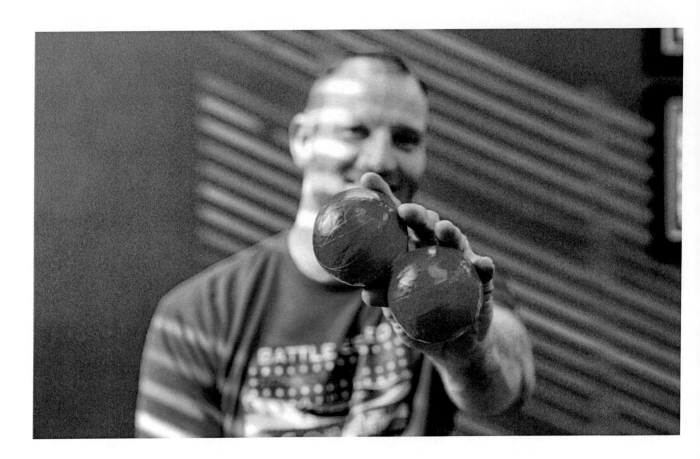

Making the BT Peanut

One of the SMR/Recovery tools we use the most is the BT Peanut. Everything else you need for the corrective protocols on the following pages can be purchased at a sporting goods store. A peanut might be harder to find. The good news is, they are very easy to make!

Take two T-balls (soft core baseballs that little kids hit off a T) and a roll of electrical tape. Hold the balls together while you tape them to each other and start wrapping. Be sure to transition frequently from one ball to the next. The more times you cross over, the sturdier the peanut will be. Also, be sure to wrap the sides equally. A peanut with one side bigger than the other is uncomfortable to use and doesn't promote postural balance! Keep wrapping until you can no longer see any of the T-ball between the tape. I usually use an entire roll of tape for one peanut. T-balls are nice because they have a little bit of give. Regular baseballs can also be used for more pressure.

Corrective Protocol 1 - Feet and Lower Leg

       This protocol is designed to address lower leg issues such as shin pain, calf tightness and pain, heel and foot pain. Posturally, it can be used to address collapsing arches, poor ankle mobility, and poor knee mobility. We will work from the ground, up, starting by rolling the bottom of the foot, then working up the lower leg, and finally the posterior knee.

*Bouncy Ball or Barbell Foot Roll	Roll 30-60 seconds each foot
*Foam Roll Calves	Roll 30-60 seconds each calf
Foam Roll Shins	Roll 30-60 seconds together
Lacrosse Ball Shins	Work in deeper on tight spots as needed
*Tennis Ball Squat	Hold 30 seconds 1-2 spots per leg
*Gravity Drop Calf Stretch	Hold for 1 minute
PNF Stretch Calves	3 x 10 seconds contract/10 seconds relax
*Toe Taps	2 x 30-60 seconds

When time is limited, you can get by with just the exercises with stars

Corrective Protocol 1 - Feet and Lower Leg

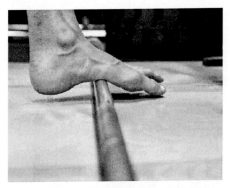

Barbell Roll Feet

This can be done sitting or standing depending how much pressure you want to apply. Slowly roll from the ball of the foot to the heel and back. Pause on the tight spots, allowing them to relax and release. This can also be done with a bouncy ball for softer, but more targeted pressure. Spend 30-60 seconds on each foot.

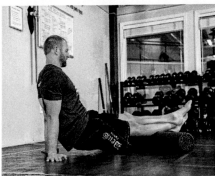

Foam Roll Calves

While sitting on the floor, place your lower legs on a foam roller. With your hands under your shoulders, lift your hips up to apply pressure to the calves. You can start with both calves on the roller. To apply more pressure, cross one leg over the other. Roll back and forth from the heel to the back of the knee. Spend 30-60 seconds on each leg.

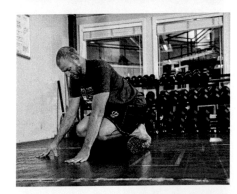

Foam Roll Shins

Begin kneeling on a foam roller while balancing yourself with your hands on the floor. Slowly roll back and forth from the knee to the ankles. Spend 30-60 seconds rolling the shins.

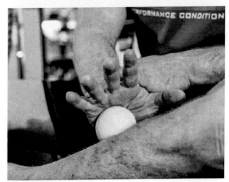

Lacrosse Ball Shins

While sitting on the floor with hip externally rotated, firmly roll a lacrosse ball along the medial side of the tibia. You can apply more pressure with your hand to address tight spots. Once you have rolled the length of the tibia, move the hip into a neutral position with the bent knee in front of you to roll along the lateral side of the tibia. Focus on the tight spots, applying firm pressure with your hand.

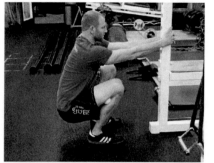

Tennis Ball Squat

Place a tennis ball behind the knee where the lateral calf and hamstring tendons cross the knee joint. While holding something for support, lower into a deep squat to smash the tennis ball in the joint. Hold this approximately 30 seconds, then move the tennis ball in to where the medial calf and hamstrings tendons cross the joint. Hold another 30 seconds here, then switch legs. This serves both to smash the tendons, releasing tension, as well as tractioning the joint itself, opening it up to increase fluid movement.

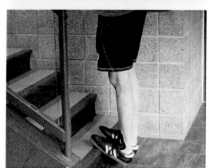

Gravity Drop Calf Stretch

Place the balls of both feet on a stair. Hold onto the stair rail to keep your entire body lined up vertically over your heels. Slowly lower your heels into a deep calf stretch. Hold this position with relaxed calves for 1 minute.

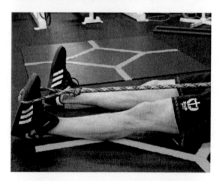

PNF Calf Stretch

Loop a recovery rope, martial arts belt, or towel around the ball of your foot. Lie down and pull on the rope to stretch your calf. While holding the stretch, attempt to plantar flex the ankle to push firmly against the rope. Hold this contraction for 10 seconds, then relax for 10 seconds while attempting to pull the ankle into an even deeper calf stretch. Repeat this cycle of contracting and relaxing for 3 rounds.

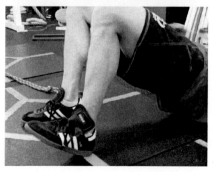

Toe Taps

While lying supine with your knees bent and feet hip width apart, bridge your hips up. Hold this position and keep your heels down while alternately tapping your toes rapidly. You will slow down as time goes, but tap as fast as possible. You should feel the tibialis anterior, or muscle on the front of your shin, will start burning. The goal is to keep going another 15-20 seconds once it starts to burn. Begin with a couple sets of 30 seconds and work up to 60 second sets.

Corrective Protocol 2 - Knees, Hips, and Lower Back

      This protocol is designed to address knee, hip, and lower back pain. Posturally, it can be used to address lower body cross syndrome which is characterized by anterior pelvic tilt, tight hip flexors and lower back, and weak gluteals and abdominals.

*Peanut Roll Quadriceps	Roll 60-120 seconds each leg
Barbell Roll Quadriceps	Roll 30-60 seconds each leg
Foam Roll Hamstrings	Roll 60-120 seconds each leg
Foam Roll IT Band	Roll 60-120 seconds each leg
*Foam Roll Low Back	Roll 30-60 seconds
*Foam Roll Sacrum	Roll 30-60 seconds
Lacrosse Ball Psoas Release	2-3 x each side
*Hip Flexor Stretch	Hold 1 minute each leg
PNF Quadriceps Stretch	3 x 10 seconds contract/10 seconds relax
*Banded 1-leg Distraction	1 minute each leg
Banded Hamstring Stretch	Hold 30-60 seconds
Banded Hip Mobility	30-60 seconds each side
*Dead Bug	3 x 15-30 seconds each side
*Stability Ball Hip Thrust	1 x 20
1-leg Hip Extension	1 x 8-12 each leg

* *When time is limited, you can get by with just the exercises with stars*

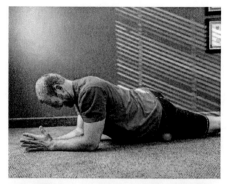

Peanut Roll Quadriceps

Start on your elbows like you are planking, but drop your hips toward the floor. Place a BT peanut just below your ASIS (anterior superior iliac spine) and slowly begin to inch your body slowly forward, allowing your weight to drive the peanut into your superficial and lateral quads. Your hips should be slightly rotated into the peanut. One side of the peanut should separate the vastus lateralus and IT band, and the other should come right down the middle of the rectus femoris. Work your way slowly from hip to knee.

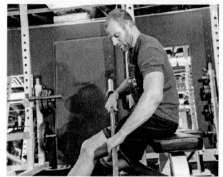

Barbell Roll Quadriceps

A barbell will work even deeper into the quads than a peanut will. Begin by sitting on a bench with the leg you are about to work extended forward. Start at the tensor fascia latae, just below the ASIS (anterior superior iliac spine) and slowly roll down the length of your quads, angling the bar both directions to get the central, medial and lateral quads. Roll slowly, pausing on tight spots to allow them to release before moving on. Spend however long it takes to go the length of your quads.

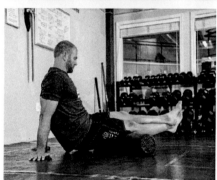

Foam Roll Hamstrings

Begin by sitting on the foam roller, with your hands behind you to hold yourself up. Cross one leg over the other to apply most of the pressure to one leg, then slowly roll back and forth from the hamstring attachment on the pelvis to the back of the knee. Spend 30-60 seconds on each leg.

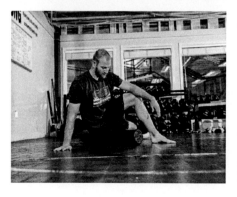

Foam Roll IT Band

Begin in the hamstring rolling position, but then cross one leg over the other and rotate your hips to place your lateral thigh on the foam roller. Roll slowly from the greater trochanter of the femur (the big, bony knob at the top of the leg near the hip) down to the lateral knee. Spend 30-60 seconds on each leg. This will likely be extremely uncomfortable. The IT band is primarily tendon, so don't expect it to loosen up as much as the quadriceps or hamstrings. You will know it is working if rolling the IT bands gets less painful from session to session.

Corrective Protocol 2 - Knees, Hips, and Lower Back

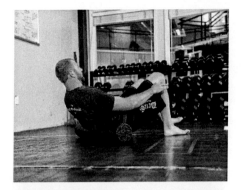

Foam Roll Low Back

Rolling the low back is somewhat controversial. This is for a couple of reasons. One, it is possible to injure a floating rib by applying too much pressure there. Two, because the lumbar spine is not supported by ribs, the vertebrae are somewhat less stable and more susceptible to disk injuries. That being said, if you crunch up slightly to engage the anterior core, the lumbar spine will be stabilized. This also elongates the spinal erectors while you are rolling them, which can be very effective in reducing low back tightness.

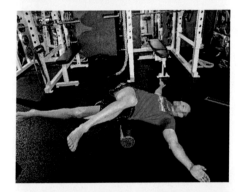

Foam Roll Rotation Sacrum

Tightness around the sacrum and through glute medius and glute minimus can contribute greatly to low back pain, limited hip mobility, and general hip tightness. For this technique, lay on the floor with your sacrum directly on the roller. As with rolling the low back, contract your anterior abdominals to stabilize the lumbar spine before you begin.

Once in position, slowly rotate your hips from side to side, allowing the roller to open up space between the greater trochanter of the femur and the crest of the ilium (broad, rounded bone at the top of the pelvis). I bend the knee of the leg coming across, while extending the bottom leg that is in contact with the roller. Roll back and forth for 30-60 seconds.

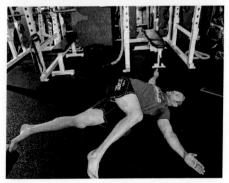

Lacrosse Ball Psoas Release

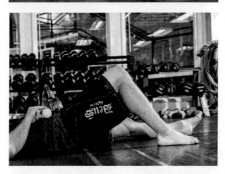

The psoas is deep abdominal muscle that runs from the lumbar spine to the inner side of the upper femur. The psoas has various attachments from T12-L5 and on the lesser trochanter of the femur. This means when the psoas is tight, it actually pulls forward on the lumbar spine, contributing to low back and pelvic positioning issues.

It is best to have a trained therapist release your psoas, but in a pinch, here is an alternative SMR technique from Kelly Starrett's book, *Becoming a Supple Leopard*. While we often do most correctives prior to lifting, Kelly cautions not to do mobilizations that may alter spinal mechanics prior to heavy lifting. Feel free to do this before most workouts, however, if you are planning to do heavy dead-lifts or squats, you should play it safe and save this for after the workout.

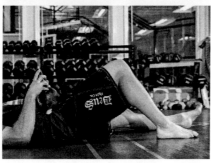

Begin on your back with the knee bent on the side you will be releasing. If you bend both knees, this release will be less intense, so you may choose to begin that way. Place a lacrosse ball roughly midway between your ASIS (anterior superior iliac spine) and your navel, just lateral of the rectus abdominus or 6-pack muscles. Set a medium-sized kettlebell on the lacrosse ball and apply more pressure with hands as needed.

From this starting position, slowly slide your foot out (keeping it in contact with the ground) until your leg is straight. When your leg is straight, slowly slide your foot back to the starting position. You may also play around with rotating the hip in and out both prior to extending the leg and once the leg is straight.

One or two times per side is usually sufficient for this technique. Remember, the slower you go, the more tolerable this technique will be.

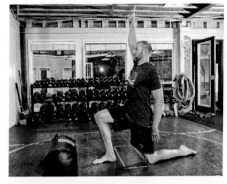

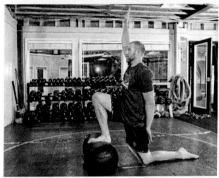

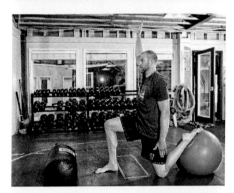

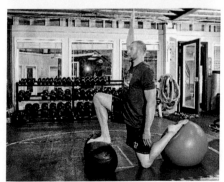

Hip Flexor Stretch

There are several progressions we like to use to a basic hip flexor stretch. First and foremost, it is important to hold up the arm opposite that shown in the photographs. Pretty sure that's what happens when you try to hurry through photographs.

Begin in a half kneeling position. Be sure to maintain a neutral lumbar spine while driving the hips forward to stretch the hip flexors on the rear leg. If you allow the lumbar spine to arch, it tilts the pelvis forward, minimizing the stretch on the hip flexors. Hold this stretch for one minute on each side.

Elevating the front foot, either on a heavy bag or a 6-12" plyometric box opens up the rear hip even more, putting the hip flexors on even greater stretch.

To emphasize the stretch on the quadriceps (rectus femoris, which is the most superficial quad muscle, is also a hip flexor), flex the rear foot more by elevate the rear foot, either on a stability ball or on a bench.

The final progression is to elevate both the front foot and the rear foot. Remember to keep a neutral lumbar spine to maintain maximal hip flexor stretch. Hold for one minute each side.

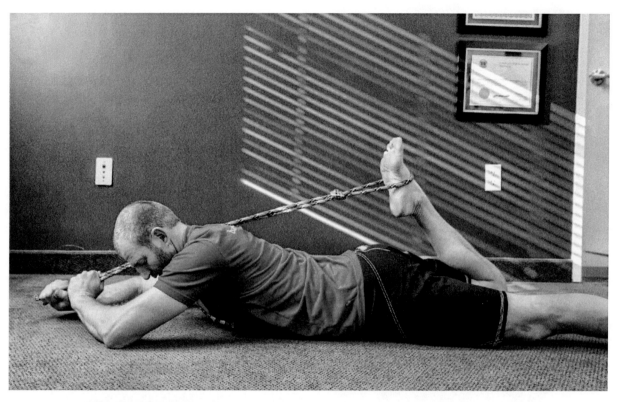

PNF Quadriceps Stretch

Propioceptive Neuromuscular Facilitation (PNF) is a quick, simple way to increase range of motion and get a deeper stretch. It relies on the golgi tendon organ (GTO) to release neurological guarding. The GTO is a neuroreceptor in the muscle that protects the muscle from contracting too hard and tearing by relaxing the muscle when it is contracting against something it cannot move. When you resist the movement, then relax into the stretch, the GTO releases the muscle tension, allowing for a greater stretch.

Lay prone (face down) with your SMR rope, a belt, or a towel around one foot. With the end of the rope or other tool, pull your heel toward your glutes until you feel a decent stretch in your quads. While resisting the movement, push back towards the floor, attempting to extend the knee. Hold this tension for 10 seconds, then relax and pull the stretch slightly further. Repeat this sequence 3 times, attempting to pull the stretch further each time you relax. Switch legs and repeat.

Corrective Protocol 2 - Knees, Hips, and Lower Back

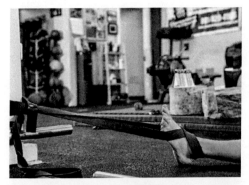

Banded 1-Leg Distraction

This is a great distraction technique for the ankle, knee, hip, and low back.

Attach a 2" superband to a squat rack or another immoveable object fairly close to the ground. Loop the band around your heel, then bring the band over the ankle, making an X on the top of the foot.

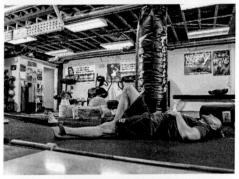

Keep the banded leg straight and relaxed, while using the bent, other leg to push backward away from the band attachment, applying more tension. Hold this position for 2 minutes, then switch the band to the opposite leg and repeat.

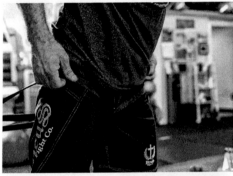

Banded Hamstring Stretch

Attach two 1" superbands to a squat rack at slightly lower than hip height. Facing away from the band attachments, loop each band around a leg and slowly walk out until there is tension on the bands. Hinge over at the hips and reach down to place the hands on the floor.

Once the hands are on the floor, squeeze the shoulder blades together and attempt to pull the chest and head toward the legs to stretch the hamstrings. Hold this position for one minute.

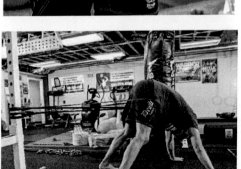

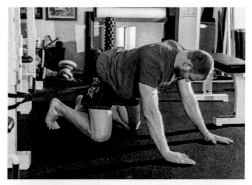

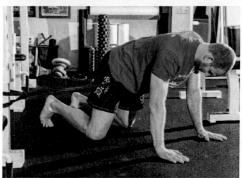

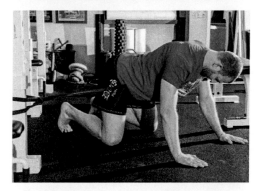

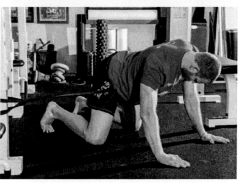

Corrective Protocol 2 - Knees, Hips, and Lower Back

<u>Banded Hip Mobility</u>

This is a great exercise to use as a corrective for hip and low back issues, as well as for a general warm-up prior to doing squats or lunges. The purpose of the movement is to traction the hip, pulling the head of the femur away from the acetabulum, allowing for more freedom of movement during the exercise.

Begin with a 1" superband attached to a squat rack or other immoveable object. Loop the other end of the band around the upper thigh as high up as possible (ideally across the lesser trochanter of the femur).

Start on hands and knees with band tension pulling the femur laterally. From this position, gently rock hips forward and backward a dozen times, then from side to side a dozen times.

Switch legs and repeat the same movements on the opposite side.

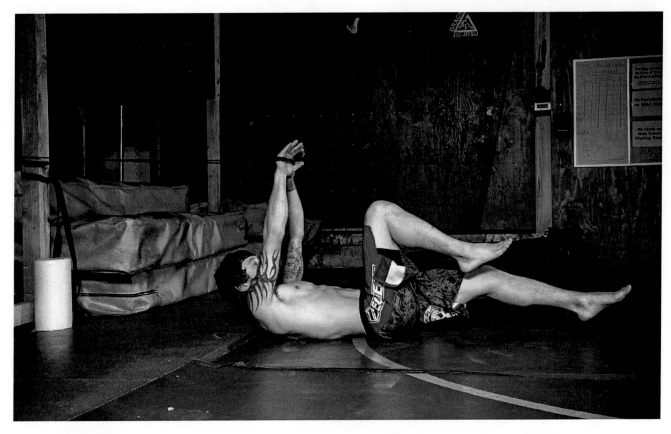

Dead Bug

One of the primary concerns we see with hip and low back issues is weak abdominals, and specifically the transverse abdominus, a deep lumbar stabilizer. The dead bug is a fantastic exercise to engage the transverse abdominus to increase lumbar stability. It's quite common for a seemingly strong athlete to struggle to keep his low back against the floor without shaking uncontrollably after 15 seconds.

For the basic dead bug, begin on your back with your right arm extended above your head and right leg extended slightly above the floor. Hold your left arm by your side, but off of the mat, and your left leg also up, with the knee bent. Keep your lower back pressed firmly against the floor, and your shoulder blades off of the floor. Focus on not letting the rectus abdominus (six pack muscles) take over the movement, but rather on engaging the deep transverse abdominus muscle to hold your back against the floor. Start with several sets of 15-30 seconds per side.

The banded dead bug, as pictured, is a more challenging progression of the exercise. Begin in the traditional dead bug position, but with your hands directly above your shoulders, holding tension on a resistance band. Hold statically for 15-30 seconds per side. You can also begin to incorporate movement, slowly switching leg positions back and forth without allowing the lower back to come off of the floor. When alternately switching the legs, go as long as possible until the shoulder blades touch the floor or the lumbar spine can no longer be held against the floor.

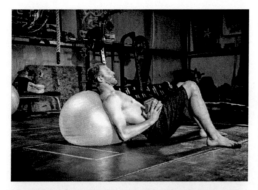

Stability Ball Hip Thrust

Begin with your head and shoulders on the stability ball with your feet shoulder width apart. Keeping a 90 degree angle at the knees, bridge your hips up as high as possible without allowing the ball to roll forward or backward. Pause at the top of the movement for two seconds, then slowly lower your hips to tap the floor. Do 20 slow and controlled repetitions, focusing on squeezing your gluteals throughout the movement. Use a dumbbell on the hips to increase resistance.

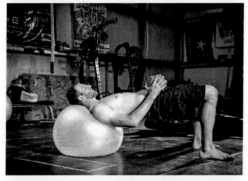

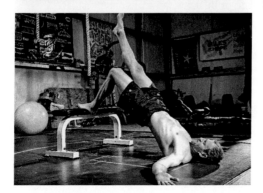

1-Leg Hip Extension

Another, slightly more demanding bodyweight exercise for the gluteals is the 1-leg hip extension. Lie on the floor with one foot on the edge of a bench. Keep the knee of this leg bent at 90 degrees. Drive through the heel to bridge up into full hip extension. Pause two seconds, and lower back to the starting position. Keep the opposite leg as close to in line with your body as possible, careful not to swing it up in effort to bring the hips up. Perform 8-12 repetitions on one leg, then switch.

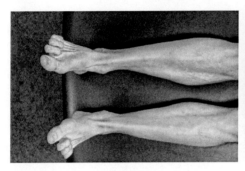
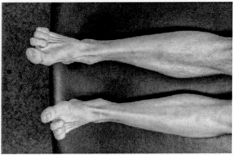

Normal sacroiliac joint - medial malleoli and heels line up directly across from each other when supine

Abnormal sacroiliac joint - medial malleoli and heels do not line up across from each other when supine

Sacroiliac (SI) Joint Disfunction

SI issues are very common among athletes, especially those who run, carry heavy loads, or do martial arts. They are characterized by dull, achy pain around the sacrum, typically on one side. Pain can be made sharper with certain movements, such as lowering into squat or lumbar flexion. This pain can also be accompanied by tight, burning hip flexors, sciatic pain, one-sided hip pain, hamstring pain, achilles pain, or side stitches.

Actual SI misalignment is frequently a joint stability issue and is often a result of muscle imbalance and tight hips. Frequently sitting with the legs crossed or standing while leaning against something or putting all your weight on one side seems to increase risk. Unevenly loading the hips during grappling (like when defending the pass or sweeping with butterfly guard) can also lead to problems. Single leg impact (jumping out of a truck bed for example and landing with most of your weight on one leg) can also cause issues.

Without an actual misalignment, SI pain can be a result of cumulative load on the joint. In *Low Back Disorders*, spinal researcher Stuart McGill, PhD., writes, "The area of tendon-periosteum attachment and extensor aponeurosis is relatively small in relation to the volume of muscle in series with the tendon complex. From this, a hypothesis evolved that the seeming mismatch of large muscle tissue to small attachment area for connective tissue places the connective tissue at high risk of sustaining microfailure, resulting in pain."

A misalignment can frequently be resolved by a therapist, or by using the realignment strategy on the following page. In addition to this, perform SMR work on the tensor fascia latae (TFL), gluteus medius, piriformis and rectus femoris. Pain without misalignment can often be improved through just SMR, however, the realignment strategy can help activate lazy stabilizers.

To assess SI misalignment, lay supine with legs outstretched. If the right and left iliac crests are lined up and the medial maleoli do not line up (apparent leg length discrepancy), there is likely a SI problem.

Corrective Protocol 2 - Knees, Hips, and Lower Back

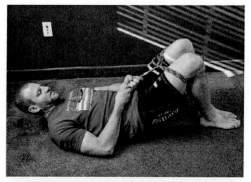

SI Realignment - Step 1

With your feet and knees together, bend your knees to draw your feet toward your glutes. Wrap your PNF rope around your legs just above the knees, pulling the straight end through the loop. Pull the rope tight enough that your knees don't come apart, then push out with your knees as hard as possible against the resistance for 5-10 seconds.

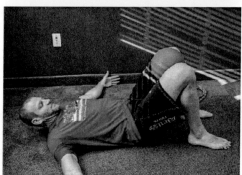

SI Realignment - Step 2

Now remove the rope, and place a medicine ball or a dumbbell between your knees. Squeeze the ball or dumbbell as hard as possible for another 5-10 seconds. You will occassionally feel or hear the SI joint slip back into place during this step.

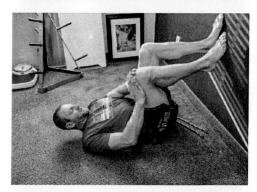

SI Realignment - Step 3

Next place your feet against the wall from a distance that your hips and knees stay flexed at approximately 90 degrees. Brace your hands against one knee, then simultaneously drive that knee against the resistance of your hands while driving the opposite foot into the wall.

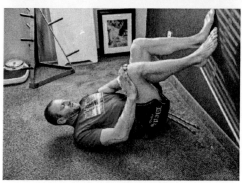

SI Realignment - Step 4

Repeat step 3 on the opposite side. You may have to go through these steps several times, checking each time if your medial malleoli align.

Corrective Protocol 3 - Upper Back and Shoulders

This protocol is designed to combat upper back pain and shoulder pain. Posturally, it addresses poor thoracic mobility, excessive kyphosis and chronically tight chest and internal rotators of the shoulder while strengthening the upper back and external rotators.

Foam Roll Upper Back	30-60 seconds
Peanut Roll Upper Back	60-120 seconds working from T1-T12
*Foam Roll Lattisimus	30-60 seconds
*MB Chest	60-120 seconds w/arm movement
Finger Pin and Stretch Chest	Work along bottom of clavicle w/arm movement
Golf Club Thoracic Rotation	Perform 5-10 rotations each side
*PVC Mobility	Perform 12-15 repetitions
*PNF Shoulders	3 x 10 seconds contract/10 seconds relax
Banded Shoulder Distraction	Hold 30-60 seconds
*Scapular Wall Slide	Perform 5-10 repetitions
*Band Pull-apart	Perform 12-15 repetitions
Vertical Band Pull-apart	Perform 12-15 repetitions
Abducted Shoulder External Rotation	Perform 12-15 repetitions
Isometric Shoulder Abduction	Hold 30 seconds

When time is limited, you can get by with just the exercises with stars

Corrective Protocol 3 - Upper Back and Shoulders

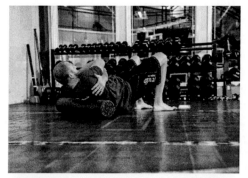

Foam Rolling the Upper Back

Begin laying face up with our upper back across a foam roller. With the roller perpendicular to your spine, cross your arms over your chest to open up your shoulder blades. Bridge your hips off the floor and slowly roll the thoracic spine, from the base of the neck to mid back. The higher your hips, the more pressure you can apply. Roll up and down the spine, pausing on tight, painful spots allowing them to release.
Be cautious not to apply too much pressure to the 12th rib. Roll 30-60 seconds.

Peanut Roll the Upper Back

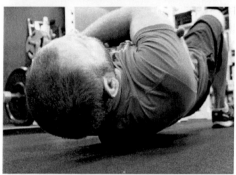

Begin with the roller at the base of your neck. I like to center C7 in in center groove of the peanut and make this my starting point. Rather than rolling back and forth, make one really slow pass from T1-T12, trying to feel the pressure at each vertebral level, pausing for a several seconds between each vertebrae. Similar to the foam roller, if you lift your hips higher, you can apply more pressure.

Foam Roll Lats

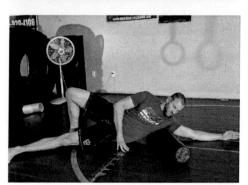

With shoulder abducted to expose the lat, lay on your side across the roller. Extend the bottom leg and keep the top knee bent with foot down to help move your body across the roller. Slowly roll from the upper portion of the triceps muscle, down the side, nearly to the bottom of the rib cage. Pause on tight, painful spots allowing them to release. Roll 30-60 seconds on each side.

Corrective Protocol 3 - Upper Back and Shoulders

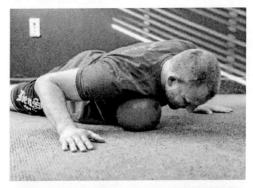

Medicine Ball Chest Release

Begin laying face down with your chest on a small firm medicine ball. The ball should be just below the collar bone. Applying pressure to the pectoral muscles, slowly roll side to side and up and down to work the upper chest. On tight, painful spots, pause to pin down the restricted area and slowly slide your hand up and down, taking the shoulder you are treating through its range of motion to allow the muscle to allow the restricted areas to release. A softball will also work for this. Roll 30-60 seconds each side.

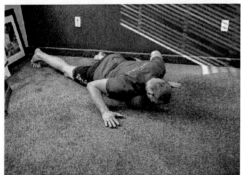

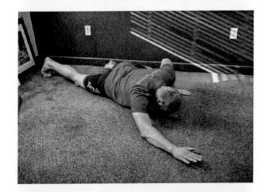

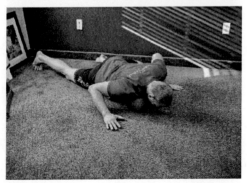

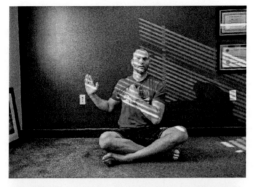

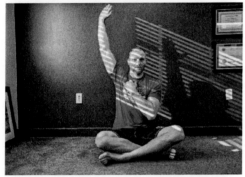

Corrective Protocol 3 - Upper Back and Shoulders

Finger Pin and Stretch

Bring one hand up by your shoulder. With the other hand, keep stiff, nearly straight fingers to apply firm pressure to the pectoral attachments on the inferior clavicle. Trace the bottom of the collarbone, with the fingers, applying , pressure then raising the hand toward the ceiling and back down, taking the shoulder through it's range of motion. Begin right next to the sternum and work your way laterally. Once you have gone the entire length of the clavicle, revisit the areas of most restriction. When you have completed one side, repeat on the other side of the chest.

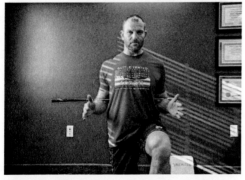

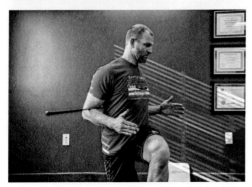

Golf Club Thoracic Rotation

This exercise can be a good assessment tool as well as a good corrective stretch in case of limited range of motion. Begin in a half kneeling position with a golf club behind your back, in the bend of your elbows. Slowly rotate toward the front leg, while not allowing the club to lose contact with either latisimus muscle and while not allowing the front knee to drift laterally past the front foot. Once you reach the point you can no longer turn without the club coming off the rear lat, pause, and return to start. Repeat 5-10 times each side.

Corrective Protocol 3 - Upper Back and Shoulders

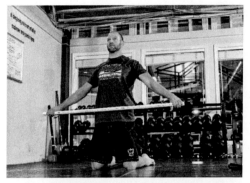

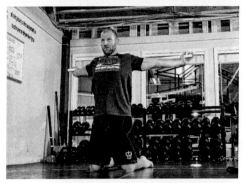

PVC Shoulder Mobility

With hands wide, begin by holding a small piece of PVC pipe in both hands. Keep your elbows straight and bring the PVC over your head and behind your back. The goal is to bring the PVC back far enough that you are actually touching it to your low back or glutes. You want there to be a definite stretch, but don't force the movement if you are struggling to get the PVC overhead. The further out your hands are, the easier the movement. If the movement is too easy, slide your hands closer together. Adjust your hands until you are able to make the complete range of motion, feeling a good stretch while transitioning overhead but are still able to keep the movement smooth. Repeat for 12-15 repetitions

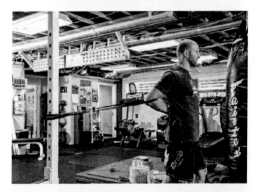

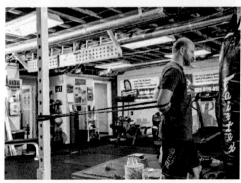

PNF Shoulder Stretch

Stand with a 1" superband attached behind you and looped around the bend of your elbow, pulling it backward. If the band is around your right elbow, place the back of your right hand against your sacrum and support it with your opposite hand. Keeping your right hand in place, press your elbow forward against the tension of the band for 10 seconds. After 10 seconds of contracting against resistance, relax for 10 seconds, allowing the band to pull your elbow (and therefore shoulder as well) backward. Continue contracting and relaxing for 3-4 times each, then switch arms. Each time that you relax, inch your feet slightly forward to increase the pull of the band.

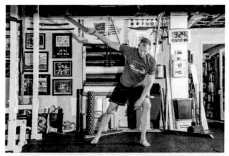

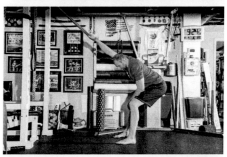

Banded Shoulder Distraction

Begin with a 2" superband attached high on a squat rack, or other immoveable object. Stick your hand through the band from the bottom, then grasp the band with your hand. Step far enough from the rack that there is tension on the band. From here, begin to lean away from the band at different angles, tractioning the shoulder joint for 10-20 seconds before shifting to a different position. Spend 60-90 seconds on each arm.

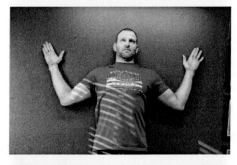

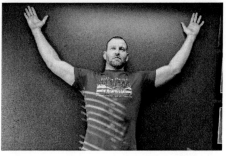

Scapular Wall Slide

Begin with your feet approximately 18 inches away from a wall, with your shoulder blades, elbows, forearms, and wrists flat against a wall. Slowly begin raising your arms up, overhead while keeping all parts of the arms against the wall. As soon as an elbow, wrist, or any other part of the arm can no longer be kept in contact with the wall, switch directions and begin pulling the elbows down towards the sides. Perform 5-10 slow repetitions.

Corrective Protocol 3 - Upper Back and Shoulders

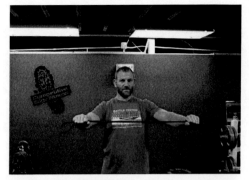

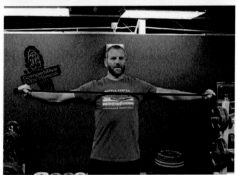

Band Pull-apart

Begin with a 1/2" to 1" superband. Depending on the strength of the band, hold it in front of you with your hands at shoulder width, or slightly wider. The further apart your hands are, the easier the exercise will be. While keeping arms straight, squeeze your shoulder blades together and pull your hands apart to bring the band against your chest. Eccentrically return to the starting position. Repeat for 12-15 repetitions.

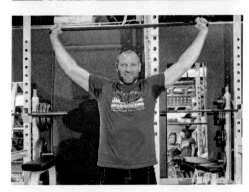

Vertical Band Pull-apart

Begin with a 1/2" to 1" superband. Depending on the strength of the band, hold it overhead with your hands at shoulder width, or slightly wider. The further apart your hands are, the easier the exercise will be. While keeping arms straight, squeeze your shoulder blades together and down while pulling your hands apart to bring the band behind your back to your shoulders. Eccentrically return to the starting position. Repeat for 12-15 repetitions.

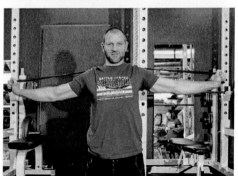

Corrective Protocol 3 - Upper Back and Shoulders

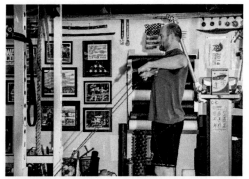

Abducted External Shoulder Rotation

Begin with a light resistance band around a low anchor point (squat rack or bench). While facing the anchor, abduct your shoulders to bring the elbows up laterally to shoulder height. From this position, with the hands also at shoulder height and elbows at 90 degrees, externally rotate the shoulders to bring the hands up overhead. Return to starting position. Perform 12-15 repetitions.

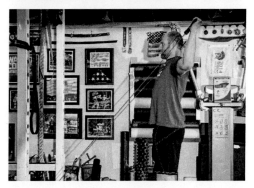

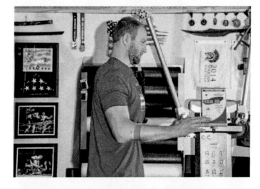

Isometric Shoulder Abduction

Begin with a mini band around the forearms near the elbows and elbows at your sides and bent at approximately 90 degrees. From this position, bring forearms out laterally 30-45 degrees. Without tensing the neck and elevating the shoulder blades, hold this position isometrically for 30 seconds.

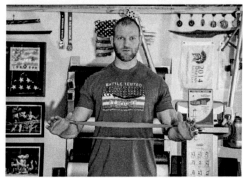

Corrective Protocol 4 - Neck

This protocol is designed to address issues such as neck stiffness and headaches. Posturally, it can be used to address head forward posture loss of lordotic curve, and cervical rotation.

*Peanut Roll Neck	Slowly roll segment by segment from C1-C7
SCM Pinch	Work from the bottom to the top of SCM
*PNF Neck Stretches (extension/rotation)	3 x 10 seconds contract/10 seconds relax
*Banded Distraction	Relax in traction 3-5 minutes
*Chin Tucks	Perform 10-15 repetitions
Banded Isometrics	Hold 10-30 seconds from multiple angles

* When time is limited, you can get by with just the exercises with stars

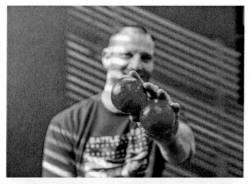

Peanut Roll Neck Extensors

Begin lying supine with the peanut at the base of the skull. Relax your head and neck completely, and slowly roll down the neck, segment by segment from C1-C7. It is also beneficial to continue rolling down the thoracic spine.

A slightly more advanced version of this is to pause at each segment to slowly flex and extend the neck. After each flexion and extension, relax again and roll slowly to the next vertebral segment.

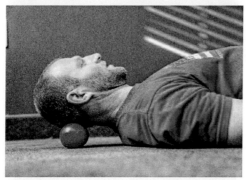

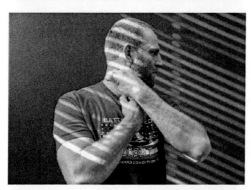

Sternocleidomastoid (SCM) Pinch

The SCM is a muscle that runs from the clavicle to the mastoid process behind the ear. When it is tight, it pulls the head forward, shortening the distance between the medial clavicle and the mastoid process. If the SCM is tight only on one side of the neck, this can also cause cervical rotation.

To begin, turn the head to bring the mastoid process and medial clavicle closer together. This will the SCM to protrude and be grasped between the index finger and the thumb. Grasp and pinch the SCM with both hands. Then, slowly move your hands back and forth in opposite directions. This is a massage technique known as breaking. Slowly work from the bottom attachment of the SCM on the clavicle upward the length of the muscle, up to the mastoid process. You may encounter trigger points, or tight, painful spots on the muscle that refer pain when you press on them. Spend extra time on these spots with firm, pulsing pressure until they release.

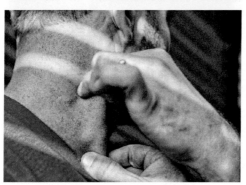

Corrective Protocol 4 - Neck

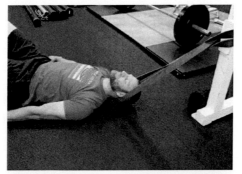

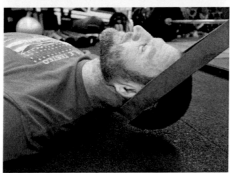

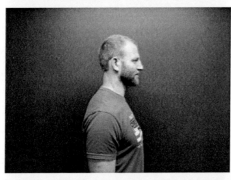

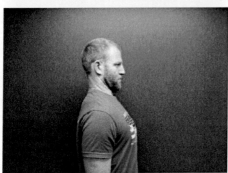

Banded Distraction

Cervical traction is something you should ask your doctor or physical therapist about before attempting. I have included it because of the tremendous relief it can provide to someone with certain neck issues. Neck problems are extremely common among fighters, so I feel it is essential to cover. By providing a gentle stretch, you can manually pull the vertebrae apart to relieve disk and neck compression. For someone with pinched nerves (often causing pain, numbness, or tingling that radiates down the arm) traction is great because it also takes pressure off of the spinal nerves.

There are a wide variety of professional and home model traction units, from inflatable pillows, to pulleys, to pneumatic devices that cost several hundred dollars. Using a superband isn't the best option, but is a cheap, practical way to try it out. Attach one end of a 1-2" superband to the squat rack about 18" up. Place the other end just below the base of the skull and lay just far enough from the rack to provide gentle tension on the band. To stay in place, the band will likely have to cover your ears. Try to relax completely and allow the band to support your head.

Chin Tucks

Begin by standing with your normal posture. Slowly pull your head back to make a double chin, being careful not to extend or flex your cervical spine. Pause for 2-3 seconds with your chin pulled back, then relax into your normal posture again. Perform 10-15 repetitions. It can be beneficial to stand with your back against a wall. This can create an additional cue to pull the back of your head toward the wall.

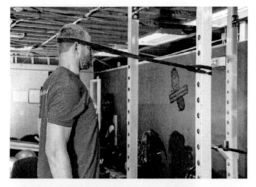

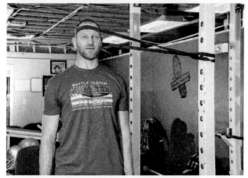

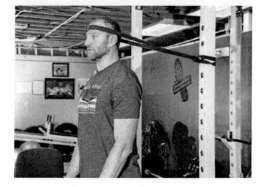

Banded Isometrics

Attach a 1" superband to a squat rack, at about chin height. Loop the band around the back of your head just above the ears and walk backward to apply tension. Your goal is to keep a neutral cervical spine regardless of the amount of pressure pullng on it. Move around a bit, rotating against the direction of the pull so that the tension shifts from pulling your head forward, to pulling sideways, to pulling backward, all while stabilizing your cervical spine against the multi-directional movement. Hold 10-30 seconds each position, or continually move for 30-60 seconds.

Corrective Protocol 5 - Hands, Forearms, and Elbows

This protocol is designed to address issues such as elbow and wrist pain.

Extensor Pin and Stretch	Roll 30-60 seconds each arm
Barbell Forearm Flexor Smash	Roll 30-60 seconds each arm
Barbell Triceps Smash	Roll 30-60 seconds each arm
Static Extensor Stretch	Hold 30-60 seconds each arm
Static Flexor Stretch	Hold 30-60 seconds each arm
Static Biceps Stretch	Hold 30-60 seconds each arm

* Do all of these if you are experiencing elbow and wrist pain.

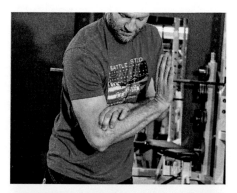
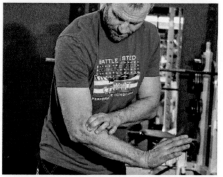
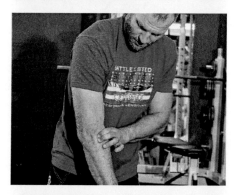
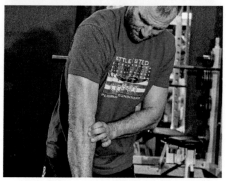

Corrective Protocol 5 - Hands, Forearms, and Elbows

Extensor Pin and Stretch

The wrist extensors come together to share one tendon, the common extensor tendon, which attaches to the lateral epicondyl of the humerus. With so many little muscles of the forearm all attaching at one relatively small point, the elbow takes a beating. Lateral epiconylitis, or tennis elbow, is a fairly common issue for people who use their hands and wrists a lot.

It is not very easy to massage the extensor muscles on your own, but you can use a technique known as Pin and Stretch. The idea is that you shorten the muscle, apply pressure on various spots along the muscle, and then lengthen the muscle while pinning a portion of it down. This is a great way to focus the stretch, targeting restrictions and adhesions that need to be broken up.

For the extensor muscles, begin by bending your elbow and extending your wrist. With your opposite hand, pin down the muscles with firm pressure near the upper attachment point. By extending your wrist you will feel the contraction of the muscles and can determine where they start. Once you have the muscle pinned down, reverse the movement, extending your elbow and flexing your wrist. This will likely be uncomfortable, but that is a good sign that you are in the right place. Take the elbow and wrist joints through their complete range of motion a couple of times, then move your hand slightly to pin down another section of the muscles. Gradually work your way down the forearm, focusing on tight, sore spots.

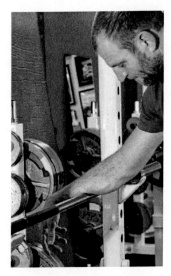

Start with simply rolling the length of the wrist flexors.

Barbell Forearm Flexor Smash

As with the wrist extensors, the wrist flexors come together to share the common flexor tendon. This tendon attaches to the medial epicondyl and is the site of medial epicondylitis, or golfers elbow. The flexors are frequently stronger and more developed than the extensors, making them a little more difficult to pin and stretch.

Instead, we use a barbell on a bench press or squat rack to first massage, then pin and stretch. Start with the barbell set at a height approximately even with your abdomen. With your hand palm down, apply pressure down into the barbell. Slowly roll or slide your forearm across the smooth, un-gnurled portion of the bar with as much pressure as you can handle working your way from wrist to elbow and back a couple of times. Once you have done this, you can begin to pin and stretch. Start near the wrist with wrist flexed and relaxed. Apply pressure and slowly extend the wrist. Move an inch or so down the forearm and repeat, continuing to pin a section of the forearm flexors down while taking the wrist through complete range of motion. After 30-60 seconds, switch arms and repeat.

Progress to pinning down portions of the muscles and taking the wrist through it's range of motion.

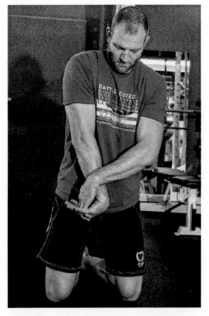

Static Extensor Stretch

The set-up for this stretch is a bit awkward, but the benefit is absolutely worth it. If you are going to stretch the wrist extensors of the right forearm, begin by holding your right arm down in front of you, then rotating your hand counter-clockwise until your thumb is pointing at your body. Then reach across your right arm with your left arm, rotate your left hand clockwise and interlock fingers. Now that your fingers are interlaced, keep your right elbow straight and pull up with your left hand. You should feel the stretch through the right forearm. Hold for 30-60 seconds and switch sides.

This can get a little confusing, so just remember that if both thumbs are pointed toward you with the fingers interlocked, the arm on the bottom is the one you are stretching.

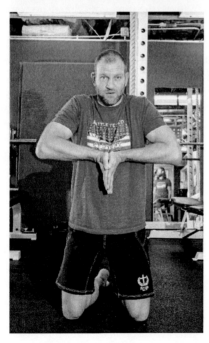

Static Flexor Stretch

This stretch is significantly easier. With your arms down, place your palms together. Slowly bend your elbows to pull your hands up toward your chest. Your elbows will point directly out to the sides as you pull your hands up. From here, you can push your fingers from one side to the other to intensify the stretch on the arm you are pushing against. Hold this stretch for 30-60 seconds.

PART III
Exercise Selection

"You've only got time for 1 lift in your program? You should deadlift. You've got time for a 2nd lift? Add chins. You can do 3 lifts? Add military presses or some form of heavy pushup. If you can do a 4th lift, don't worry about it — you're already ahead of 95% of people who lift weights" – Charles Staley

    I have always felt, if limited to three exercises, they would be the dead-lift, the push-up, and the pull-up. Each of these exercises requires heavy core involvement, and the combination of the three works all the major muscle groups. In short, these three exercises give you the most bang for your buck. As many military PT tests include push-ups and pull-ups, this gives us further reason to spend a lot of time on variations of these exercises and include them in our Battle Tested assessment. Because the sit-up is also a fundamental part of military and law enforcement tests, we will also include a variation we call the combat sit-up, a more practical variation used also to drill grappling skills. A combat sit-up flows right into a kimura, guillotine, and a sweep. In all honesty, I feel sit-ups and crunches are very over-used and this overuse can be potentially dangerous (from a spinal health standpoint). Therefore, if we are going to train them, it had better serve a greater purpose than core strength and endurance. In my experimentation, the max combat sit-up for a person, correlates closely with their regular sit-up max, so by testing the combat sit-up will give a good idea where a tactical athlete is at on the sit-up as well. Everyday will also include core strength without sit-ups. From a MMA viewpoint, bodyweight calisthenics such as push-ups, pull-ups, and sit-ups are also viewed as essential components of conditioning. In Mastering Jujitsu, Renzo Gracie writes that they have consistently proven to be the most important form of conditioning for the jujitsu fighter. He also mentions when locked in a clinch, balance, gripping strength, and driving power are necessary. So, single-leg exercises, pull-ups, dead-lifts and tire flips will also be very beneficial for fighters.

    While variations of the above exercises are the foundation of the Battle Tested program, they are far from the only exercises included and the workouts will be far from boring. This book will include both old standbys, and exercises you have never seen. On the following pages are the primary exercises we will use, categorized under the section of the workouts that you will use them.

Warm-up
Strength/Power
Test Specific
Task Specific
Grip
Finishers

Chapter 8
The Warm-up

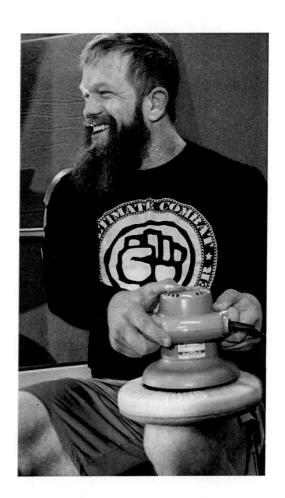

Chapter 8 – The Warm-up

The importance of a warm-up cannot be overstated. It is integral to avoiding injury and preparing the body to perform. Need evidence? A 2010 study published in the Journal of Strength and Conditioning Research showed improvement in performance in 79% of the criterions examined following a sufficient warm-up. If you could pick apart all the elements of good performance and improve 79% of those through an adequate warm-up, would you do it? Seems like a no-brainer, right? Yet many people continue to just show up and start lifting, or show up to a competition just in time to step onto the field. I'm guilty of this, and I'm sure you are from time to time as well. Why do we often cut short or even skip such an integral portion of our workout? Usually because it is uncomfortable, time consuming, and we are lazy.

A complete warm-up is much more than just heating the tissue. The goal is mobilization of the fascia. Fascia is connective tissue that surrounds everything. Each individual muscle fiber, each group of fibers, each muscle, and each group of muscles. Fascia is supposed to move freely and easily, but can get bound up and stuck. Muscular surfaces that are supposed to easily slide past each other can become tacked down and tied up on each other, restricting movement and changing movement patterns. The Battle Tested warm-up protocol includes a step-by-step process to heat this tissue, release adhesions, stretch and inhibit the hyperactive muscles, engage the underactive muscles, and get the hips and shoulders moving through their complete range of motion. This warm-up is also individualized based on your assessment in the last chapter.

1) Buffer or Warm-up
2) SMR
 3) Stretching + Correctives
4) Dynamic Movement

Following this protocol is time consuming. It will take 15-20 minutes, but is well worth the rewards of maintaining tissue health. If your life depends on staying on top of your game, it is a small price to pay. I do understand of course that you won't always have the time to do it all. Depending on the workout I'm about to complete, there are days I just use the buffer, or just do SMR, or just do the dynamic warm-up. As a general rule, the heavier you are planning to lift, or the faster you are planning to move, the more of the protocol you should complete. If you are doing a lower intensity de-load workout, or heading out for a trail run, you might get away with a short dynamic warm-up and continue to warm-up as you begin to workout. If you are intending to do sprints, or a near max lift, you should follow the entire protocol. Not only will it help your body resist injury, it will also improve movement mechanics to improve workout performance.

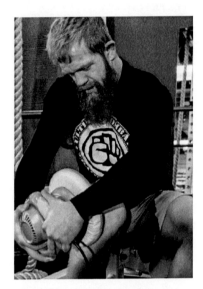

In addition to working over tight muscles, you can use the buffer directly over sore joints to address the tendons and their attachment sites.

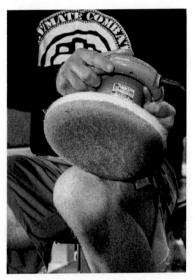

By turning the buffer and using the edge you can work deeper and target trouble spots a little better.

1) The Car Buffer

As strange as it sounds, a car buffer is a fantastic tool for warming up. Prior to doing anything else, when our athletes arrive at the gym, we recommend hitting tight, sore spots with the buffer. The forearms, calves, anterior thighs, low back, and around the sacrum are common chronically tight areas on most people that could benefit from a quick run through with the buffer. The shoulders and the chest (DO NOT buff the nipples) are also great areas to run the buffer over, but it is much easier with a smaller single hand held car buffer. Spend only a short time in each area. If an area needs further attention, work it briefly, move on, and come back to it. Leaving the buffer too long in one location will cause uncomfortable burning and tingling of the skin.

The primary purpose of the buffer is to create heat, loosening up the tissue to prepare for movement and the SMR techniques that come next in the warm-up progression. Fascia loosens and moves much easier as it heats up. This is why when you are getting a deep tissue massage, if the therapist slowly warms up the area working their way deeper and deeper, all is well. However if they immediately drive an elbow into your thigh, your muscles will freak out and respond by tensing to resist the intruding elbow.

As with the massage therapist's elbow, we will see better results by heating and loosening the area prior to diving in with a lacrosse ball or other SMR tool. In addition to heat, the vibration of the buffer also helps tissue to relax, making the fascia more receptive to SMR. In addition to creating heat, friction is also an effective way to treat scar tissue. Using the buffer on large scars can help to restore some movement, to otherwise immoble tissue.

In addition to seated general work with the buffer, I have found it very effective to incorporate range of motion through restricted movement patterns while buffing the restricted areas. A good example would be a hip hinge while buffing the lower back and glutes.

If you do not have a buffer on hand, this portion of the progression can be replaced by a short general warm-up on a rower or another less desireable cardio machine.

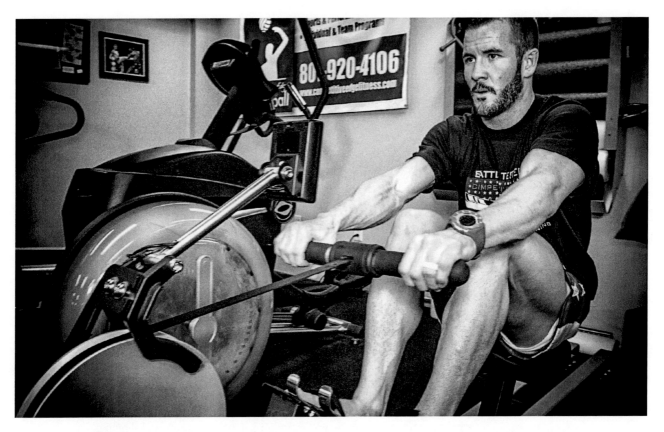

Rower

If you don't have a car buffer, or simply want to warm the tissue with something a little more dynamic, the rower is a fantastic substitute. Muscularly, the rower uses almost everything, making it a quick way to heat the entire body, preparing it for the next portion of the warm-up. The benefit of the buffer opposed to a general warm-up is that with the buffer you can begin to target tight spots from the beginning.

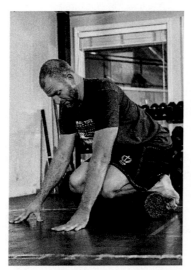

The foam roller is a great tool for general myofascial release. It is quick and easy to hit big muscles groups and large areas with a roller.

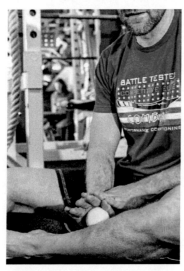

A lacrosse ball is a great tool for more targeted work to arreas that are difficult to access with a foam roller.

Self Myofascial Release (SMR)

Once the fascia is warm and loose from the buffer (or general warm-up), our efforts at self massage will work better and we will have a better shot at making lasting change in chronically tight tissue. As covered in Chapter 7, our SMR techniques can utilize foam rollers, lacrosse balls, t-balls, bouncy balls, The Stick, the Thera-cane, and even kettlebells and barbells.

The idea behind SMR is that bound up tissue can be released and mobilized by applying slow, deep pressure. Addressing these knots, or adhesions prior to your workout, you will move better and safer throughout your workout. Rather than trying to mobilize everything, SMR during the warm-up should be kept to trouble spots that are potentially restricting and altering movement patterns.

As with the buffer, common areas that need extra attention are the forearms, shoulders, chest, calves, anterior thighs and hip flexors, low back and around the sacrum. While these are definitely restrictions and imbalances that we see in a lot of athletes, the techniques used during the warm-up will differ from person to person and should be specific to you.

Look back on your assessment and see what you need to work on. The suggested techniques based on your assessment are the ones you will include in your warm-up until they are no longer an issue. Remember that the slower you go, the deeper into the tissue you will be able to penetrate, and the more likely you will be successful in releasing any adhesions.

If you have the time, it is great to address all of these issues before and after the workout. If limited to one or the other, do them here during the warm-up.

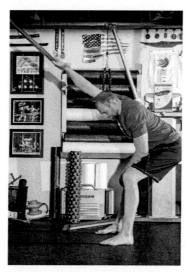

One of the fastest ways to improve flexibility, PNF stretching, uses alternating contraction and relaxation to overcome neuromuscular guarding.

Banded distraction is a great method to stretch while simultaneously gapping the joints to reduce inflammation and improve joint movement.

Stretching + Correctives

Stretching, and more specifically, static stretching, has become quite contraversial in the past 10-15 years. There is a lot of research demonstrating that static stretching temporarily decreases strength in the stretched muscles and therefore also decreases performance. I agree that it can have adverse affects, and discourage most static stretching prior to competition.

However, if I have a chronically tight, overactive muscle or muscle group, why wouldn't I want to temporarily decrease strength in this muscle prior to training? Antagonist muscles are designed to work against each other. If one is tight and shortened, the opposite is lengthened and weakened. If I have overly tight hip flexors, my pelvis will tilt anteriorly, reducing the amount of power I can produce with my hip extensors. Chronic tightness encourages misalignment and imbalances. Strength training while misaligned and imbalanced can lead to overuse injuries and worse. By addressing this imbalance during the warm-up, I can proactively work to resolve the issue.

Because a tight muscle effects both the muscle and its antagonist, it is most beneficial to address the problem from both sides. This is why we combine stretching and correctives. When I stretch my hip flexors, I am also going to activate and strengthen my hip extensors to balance out the problem. This also take advantage of the principle of reciprocal inhibition. By actively engaging the glutes, the hip flexors relax, allowing more stretch. Unfortunately, in a chronically tight muscle group, the antagonist is passively inhibited, which requires we counteract the problem through stretching and correctives.

It is hard to stretch a cold band with a knot in it. Much easier if we take time to warm up the band, then untie the knot. This is why we don't stretch until after using the buffer and releasing the knots through SMR. Once again, the particular stretches and corrective exercises that you will do for your warm-up will be dependent on the results of your assessment. Based on your assessment in Chapter 7, you will plug the recommended stretching and corrective protocols into your pre-training warm-up.

Dynamic Movement

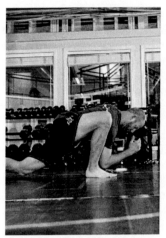

The dynamic warm-up is the final step in the complete Battle Tested warm-up. Once we have addressed the problem areas, it is time to begin taking the body through functional movements. There are many movements we can incorporate into the dynamic warm-up, ranging from general range of motion exercises to going through progressively heavier specific strength exercises prior to lifting or progressively faster sport specific movements prior to competition. When preparing to do max effort lifts, I will begin with some of the following movements and follow them with light, full range of motion practice of the lift I am going heavy on. Many of the corrective exercises from the previous chapter are also good dynamic movements, so you may already have this portion partially covered.

The following are good full body movements to take the joints through full range of motion, preparing them for loaded movement.

The World's Greatest Stretch includes hip mobility, level change, and rotation, making it a great addition to any dynamic warm-up.

Here, the Ginja Ninja, perfectly capable of squating 400+, warms up with a light set of barbell back squats at 135 lbs.

Basic Full-Body Dynamic Warm-up

World's Greatest Stretch	12 repetitions
Walking Quad Stretch	12 repetitions
Supine Knee Drop	20 repetitions
Hip Swivel	12 repetitions
Cossack Squat	12 repetitions
PVC Shoulder Mobility (page 130)	12 repetitions
Push-up	12 repetitions
Band Pull-apart (page 132)	12 repetitions

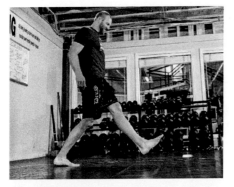

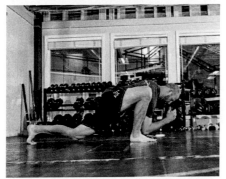

World's Greatest Stretch

I first learned this movement from Mark Verstegen's book, *Core Performance,* in which he calls it the Movement Prep Lunge. Since then I have seen a lot of people use variations of it.

Begin by taking a big step with your right foot into a lunge. Rather than staying upright, hinge over at the hips to reach the right elbow to the instep of your right foot. Place your left hand on the ground, then rotate your shoulders to the right, lifting your right arm toward the ceiling. Your knee should remain just above the floor. After the rotation, return to place both hands on the floor on each side of the right foot. With hands on the floor, drive your hips backward into a split stance hamstring stretch. Pause, holding the hamstring stretch for 2-3 seconds, then step forward with the left foot into a lunge on the opposite side. Repeat on opposite side. Continue alternating for repetitions.

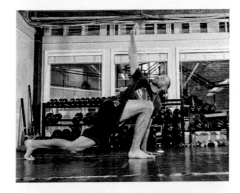

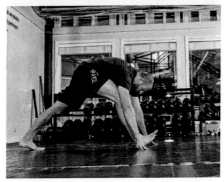

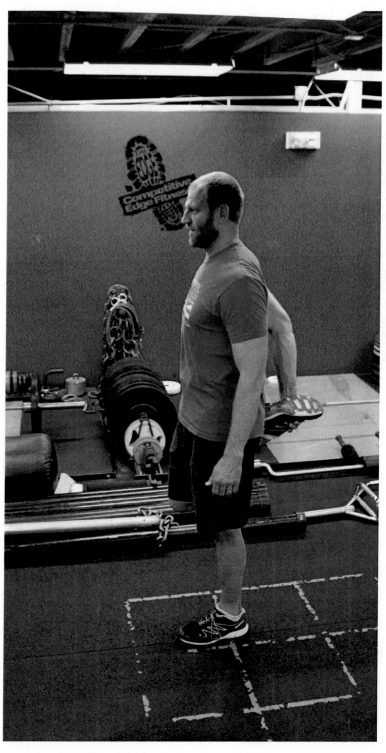

Walking Quad Stretch

The Walking Quad Stretch is similar to a standing static quad stretch. While standing, reach back to grab the top of your right ankle with your right hand. Rather than simply holding the stretch, actively pull your knee back by your ankle, while driving your hips forward. Pause long enough to raise up on the toes of the right foot, then release the ankle, take a step and repeat with the left leg. When pulling the ankle, don't let the knee drift laterally. The stretch will be better if you keep your knees close together. Perform 12 repetitions.

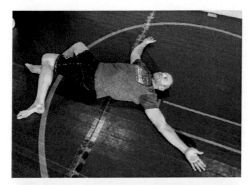

Supine Knee Drop

Begin lying flat on your back (supine) with arms outstretched to the sides, palms up, and knees bent. While keeping your shoulder blades flat on the floor and your feet approximately hip width apart, drop your knees from side to side. This movement is more hip rotation than spinal rotation. Perform 20 repetitions.

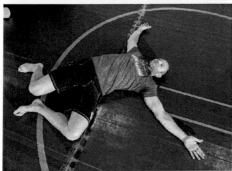

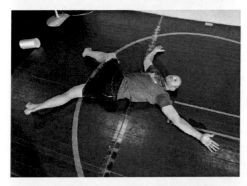

Supine Hip Swivel

Begin lying flat on your back (supine) with arms outstretched to the sides and palms up. Instead of having your knees bent, keep your legs relatively straight and rotate from side to side, reaching as far as possible with your foot. This movement is more spinal rotation than hip rotation. Perform 12 repetitions.

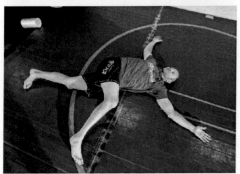

154

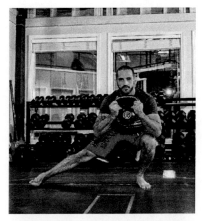

Cossack Squat

Begin the Cossack Squat with your feet nearly twice shoulder width apart. For warm-up, you can hold a light kettlebell or do it without weight. Push your hips back as if sitting in a chair as you shift your hips to the side to place your weight directly over one knee. The other leg will remain straight as you lower down. Be sure to keep your knees lined up directly over your toes. Do not allow the knee to drift laterally past the foot. If it does, try to keep your toes pointed forward and sit back more onto your heels. Pause a couple seconds, then reverse the movement, pausing again at the center start position before lowering down to the other side. Perform 12 repetitions.

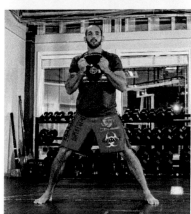

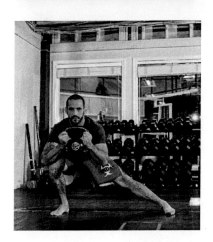

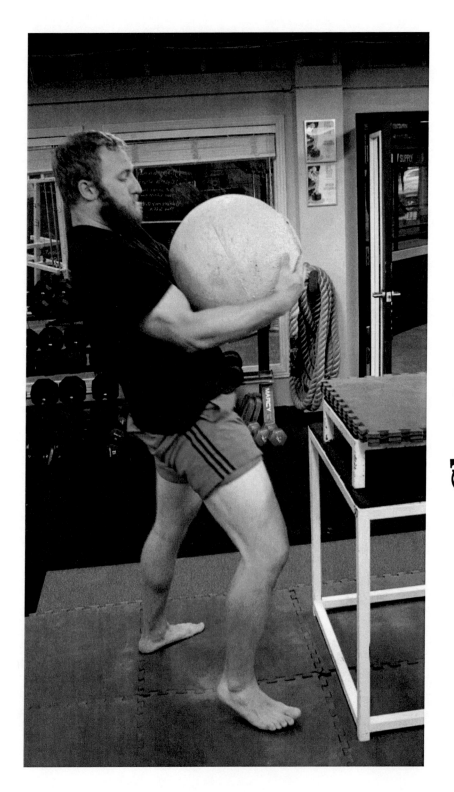

Chapter 9
Strength and Power

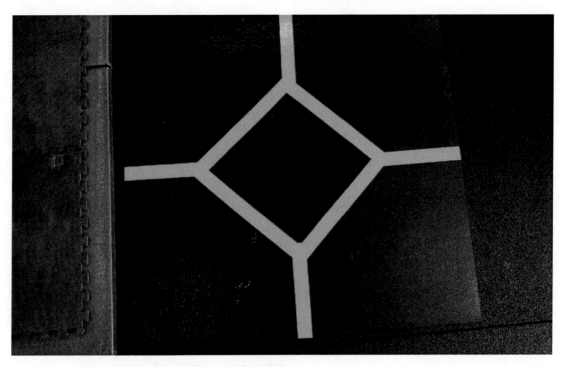

<u>Box 5 Agility Drills</u>

Session 1	2 min 40 sec
1to 4	2 x 15s
1 to 2	2 x 15s
1 to 3	2 x 15s
4 to 2	2 x 15s
1-2-3-4	1 x 20s
4-3-2-1	1 x 20s

Session 2	3 min
1-5-4-5-1	2 x 15s
1-5-2-5-1	2 x 15s
4-5-3-5-4	2 x 15s
2-5-3-5-2	2 x 15s
1 to 4	2 x 15s
1 to 2	2 x 15s

Session 3	3 min 40 sec
1 to 4	2 x 20s
1 to 2	2 x 20s
1 to 3	2 x 15s
4 to 2	2 x 15s
1-2-4-3	2 x 15s
1-4-2-3	2 x 15s
1-2-3-4-3-2-1	1 x 20s

Session 4	4 min
1-5-4-5-1	2 x 20s
1-5-2-5-1	2 x 20s
4-5-3-5-4	2 x 20s
2-5-3-5-2	2 x 20s
1 to 4	2 x 20s
1 to 2	2 x 20s

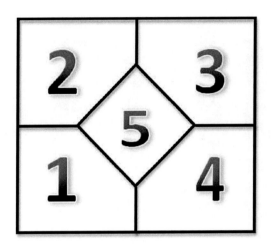

Session 5   **4 min 20 sec**

1 to 4	2 x 20s
1 to 2	2 x 20s
1 to 3	2 x 20s
4 to 2	2 x 20s
1-2-4-3	2 x 20s
1-4-2-3	2 x 20s
1-2-3-4-3-2-1	1 x 20s

Session 6   **5 min**

1-3-2-1	2 x 20s
4-2-3-4	2 x 20s
1-2-4-1	2 x 20s
4-3-1-4	2 x 20s
1-2-3-4	2 x 15s
4-3-2-1	2 x 15
1-5-2-5-3-5-4-5	2 x 20s
4-5-3-5-2-5-1-5	2 x 20s

Session 7   **5 min 20 sec**

1 to 4	2 x 20s
1 to 2	2 x 20s
1 to 3	2 x 20s
4 to 2	2 x 20s
1-2-3-4	2 x 20s
4-3-2-1	2 x 15s
2-1-4-3-4-1-2	2 x 20s
1-2-3-4-3-2-1	2 x 20

Session 8   **6 min**

1-5-4-5-1	3 x 20s
1-5-2-5-1	3 x 20s
4-5-3-5-4	3 x 20s
2-5-3-5-2	3 x 20s
1 to 4	3 x 20s
1 to 2	3 x 20s

Hip Dominant Exercises

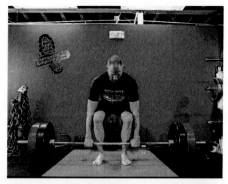

Conventional Dead-lift

For the Conventional Dead-lift, stand with feet hip width apart and your shins next to the bar. Keep your torso tall while you drop your hips back into a deep squat to grasp the barbell just outside of your knees. Squeeze your shoulder blades together and keep your back straight as you push through the floor and drive your hips forward to clear the floor. Don't hyperextend the hips at the top, but squeeze the glutes to make sure you are getting full engagement and full hip extension. Slowly reverse the movement to return the weight to the floor. While many people drop heavy weight from the top, you will become stronger if you control it with good form all the way down.

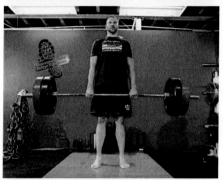

Should you use mixed grip? Only when you need to. The goal is to double overhand as long as possible. You should have two maxes - double overhand and mixed grip. Try to improve both.

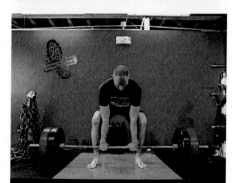

Squat Stance Dead-lift

The Squat Stance Dead-lift is just like the Conventional Dead-lift with the exception that your feet are slightly wider as they would be if you were squating. In this position, the hips are more stable and the lower back isn't taxed quite as much as it is during Conventional.

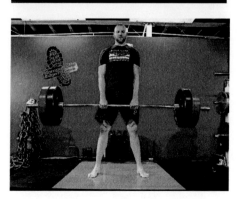

Hip Dominant Exercises

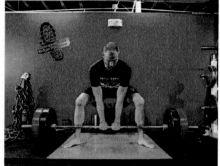

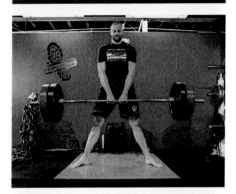

Sumo Dead-lift

The Sumo Dead-lift is another great alternative that places even more emphasis on the hips and hamstrings. Start with the feet out nearly twice shoulder width apart and toes pointed out significantly. Again, drop the hips back to lower to and grasp the bar, then push through the floor and drive your hips forward to complete the lift.

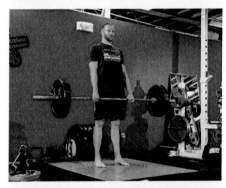

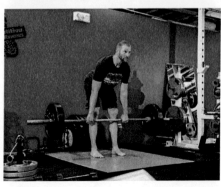

Romanian Dead-lift

This variation minimizes knee involvement and emphasizes hip movement. I like to start this movement from the top. To do this, simply perform a conventional dead-lift to reach the top position. From here, keep only a slight bend in the knees, then hinge to drive your hips backward until you get a great hamstring stretch. The bar should almost slide down your legs to the bottom position. If it does not, you are likely not pushing your hips backward far enough and you are likely putting your low back at risk for injury. Don't worry about going all the way to the floor unless your flexibility allows it. Simply lower to a good stretch, pause and squeeze your glutes to drive your hips forward to complete the movement.

Superband Dead-lift

  The most difficult portion of an exercise is the beginning of concentric contraction. This is the initial pull from the floor on a dead-lift, the bottom position of a squat, the bottom position of a bench press, etc. The closer you are to locking out,the more weight you are able to handle. That is why partial repetitions are easier than full repetitions, and why powerlifting meets have judges who enforce full depth. Adding bands to an exercise serves to make the movement more difficult at the top while keeping it manageable at the bottom. The closer you are to the top of the movement, the more the band stretches and the more resistance you have. Using bands also accelerates the eccentric or lowering phase of a movement, which in exercises like squats and bench press will lead to greater stretch reflex and more power off the bottom of the movement. Essentially, your tendons store elastic energy when being stretched which is then transfered into the contraction when the movement is reversed. Because dead-lifts start from a dead stop on the floor, the stretch reflex is negated, but occasional band use can still really be beneficial to overload lockout.

  Some lifting platforms will have pins to attach bands to, but the platforms in most regular gyms will not. Wrapping a superband around the barbell and then standing inside the ends of the band is a great alternative. The more times you wrap it around the bar, the more resistance it will provide. I usually use a 1" thick superband for dead-lifts, but play around with different bands until you find what works for you.

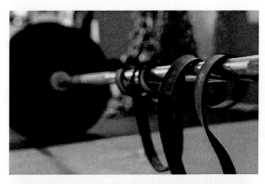
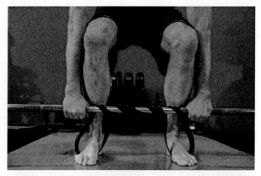
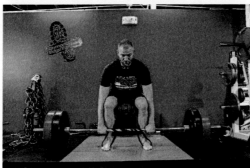
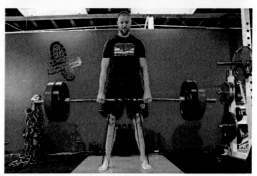

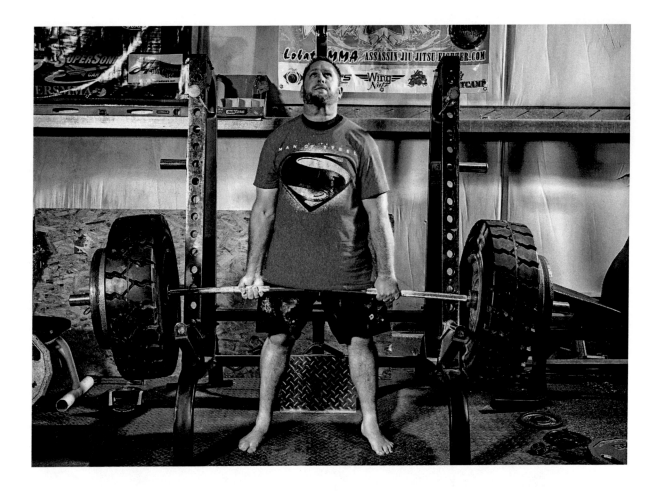

Rack Pull

The rack pull is essentially a partial range of motion dead-lift. You begin with the bar on the safety pins of a squat rack at approximately just below knee height. This eliminates the bottom portion of the dead-lift and allows you to pull from higher than the floor, in the position where you are the strongest. Because you are eliminating the hardest part of the movement, you are able to lift significantly more weight on a rack pull than you are on a dead-lift.

While this may seem counter-intuitive to take away the hard part of the movement, it serves a variety of purposes. First, it helps your body become accustomed to holding really heavy weight. A dead-lift works just about everything, and not just at the bottom. The top portion of a dead-lift, which is what you will be training with a rack pull is very challenging to grip, traps and upper back, lower back, and hips. Overloading these things with weight much greater than you are used to dead-lifting helps prep you to handle that kind of weight in the future. Secondly, rack pulls do wonders for your confidence, which is sometimes just the boost you need to hit a new PR. There is also no question that rack pulls are good for your ego.

Hip Dominant Exercises

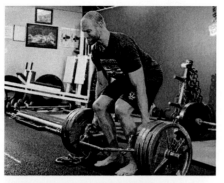

Hex Bar Dead-lift

The Hex Bar Dead-lift is similar to a Conventional Dead-ift with the exception that you are inside the bar, centering the load around your body, rather than sitting slightly in front of you. This makes the lift easier and also makes it a little more of a squat movement than the other variations.

Step into the bar, squat down to grasp the handles, squeeze the shoulder blades and simply stand up.

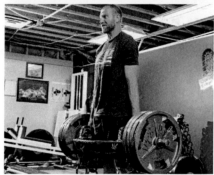

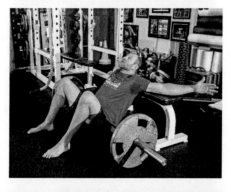

Barbell Hip Thrust

Begin with your shoulders on a bench and hips below a barbell. You may want to cushion the barbell by wrapping it in a towel or using a squat shoulder pad. Your feet should be shoulder width apart and knees should remain flexed around 90 degrees. Squeeze your glutes to bridge your hips and the barbell off of the floor. Lower slowly, focusing on controlling the movement on the way down, then explosively drive your hips into extension.

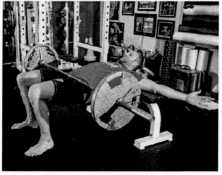

Single Leg Hip Dominant Exercises

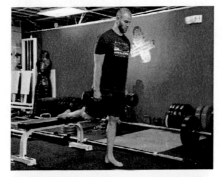

Bulgarian Split Squat

The Bulgarian Split Squat is just like a lunge, but with the rear foot elevated. Rest the top of your rear foot on the bench and place your front foot far enough forward that when you lower into the lunge, your front heel stays flat. Slowly lower your rear knee toward the floor as far as possible (this is somewhat dependent on leg length). If your front heel comes off of the floor, try bending the rear knee more, or move the front foot forward a few inches. From the bottom, focus on pushing through the heel of the front foot to return to the starting postition. Perform all repetitions on one leg before switching legs.

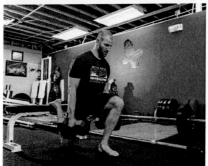

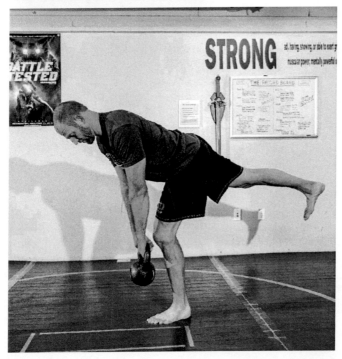

1-leg RDL

Start with a single kettlebell in both hands. Squeeze your shoulder blades together and lift one foot just off the floor. Keep a slight bend in the knee of your planted foot and hinge over at the hips to lower the kettlebell toward the floor. Keep your body straight from ear to ankle as you pivot around the planted hip. Reverse the movement when the kettlebell touches the floor or when your back starts to round, whichever comes first.

The most common mistake is to rotate the hips and allow the hip on the moving leg to turn toward the ceiling. If you focus on keeping your hips parallel to the floor and the toes pointed directly at the floor, it will help to correct this issue.

Hip Dominant Exercises

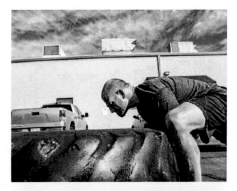

Tire Flip

Like the Dead-lift, the Tire Flip is a great full body exercise. We will classify it as a hip dominant exercise, but rest assured a big tire will work almost everything. Depending on the size of the tire, you will flip it differently. In the first picture, you will see me flipping a 335 lb. tire. For a small tire this size, you stand with your feet wide and shins and hips close to the tire. Drop your hips and get your fingers under the tire. Keep your arms fairly straight (so you don't injure your biceps) and lift the tire like you would perform a Dead-lift.

With a large tire, like the 1,250 lb. tire I am flipping in the second picture, it will be too heavy to Dead-lift. For a tire this size, you place your hip width apart quite a ways from the tire and place your chest and shoulders low on the tire. From this position, you will drive forward and upward to pivot the tire on the far edge rather than attempting to lift it.

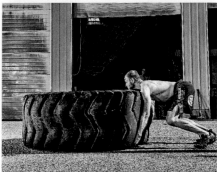

Tire Flip Variations

A fun variation with smaller tires is the Leapfrog Tire Flip. By flipping a tire over another tire, you increase the difficulty tremendously. Part of the challenge is that both tires are circular, meaning that they do not flip straight over each other, rather as you are flipping one overtop of the other, it tries to fall off the sides of the other, forcing you to fight it laterally as well to keep it from falling.

With large tires, another option is to do Team Tire Flips. You may have a tire that a single athlete can only flip 1-2 times, but if you put a couple athletes on it, they can flip it for distance or sets of 8-12.

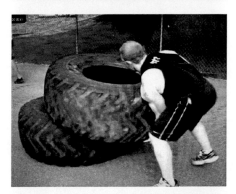

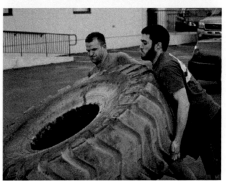

Knee Dominant Exercises

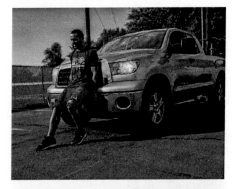

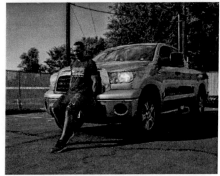

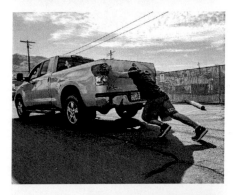

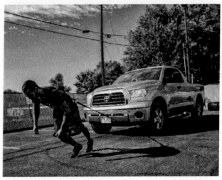

Knee Dominant Exercises

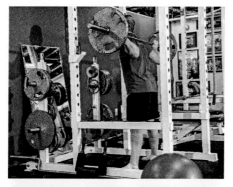

Squat

There are differing opinions of high bar or low bar squats. I honestly don't care. Do whichever is most comfortable to you as long as the bar is low enough on the traps to rest below the C7 vertebrae (the lowest vertebrae on your neck) marked by the prominent bump of the spinous process visible on the neck. Squeeze your shoulder blades together, set the bar in place and stand up under it to take it from the rack. Take a step or two backward to clear the pins before squating.

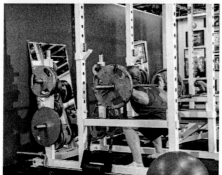

With feet slightly approximately shoulder width apart, brace your core and begin to push the hips back while maintaining a tall torso. You can expect some forward lean, just avoid letting the back round forward. As you descend, attempt to keep the angle of the spine roughly parallel to the angle of the shins. Attempt to lower until the thighs are parallel to the floor. Keep your weight on your heels, but corkscrew your feet out against the floor as you ascend to engage the glutes and keep your knees from caving in.

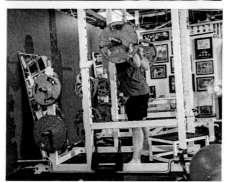

Box Squat

Box Squats are awesome for teaching correct squat mechanics, to give depth feedback and also to develop raw strength rather than stretch reflex off the bottom of the lift. We will also occassionally do High Box Squats for a variety of reasons. High Box Squats allow you to lift significantly heavier than you are capable of performing to depth. While this may be considered cheating, it also allows you as the lifter to get the feel for heavier loads on the spine as well as requiring increased muscle fiber activation.

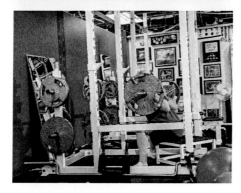

Rather than just using a high box to routinely boost our ego, we can use it as an effective way to reach new PRs. If I can squat 100 lbs. more on a 24" box than an 18" box, I can keep the weight the same as I gradually decrease the box height (1/2" to 1" per squat workout) while also increasing the weight on my 18" box squat. Eventually, I will meet in the middle with a much heavier 1 repetition max. Occassionally during this program we will superset heavy High Box Squats to increase muscle fiber activity with near max regular Squats or moderate deep Squats.

Knee Dominant Exercises

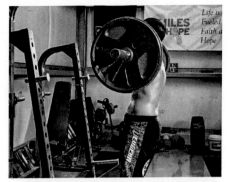

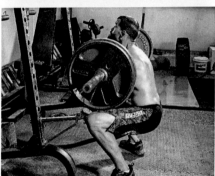

Front Squat

The Front Squat is another great variation which increases core involvement, requires more upright posture and greater shoulder mobility and strength, while emphasizing the quadriceps rather than the hips. I am terrible at front squats, but have included this link to a video where our weightlifting coach Sam will walk you through it.

Single Leg Knee Dominant Exercises

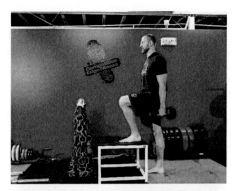

DB Step-up

Standing directly in front of an 18" plyometric box (shorter athletes may require a shorter box), place one foot, heel included, completely on the box. Lift the toes of the rear leg slightly to minimize rear leg assistance, then slowly drive through the heel of the front foot to stand up onto the box. You may place the second foot on the box only if necessary to catch your balance. Otherwise, we want to keep the entire load entirely on the working leg for the duration of the exercise..

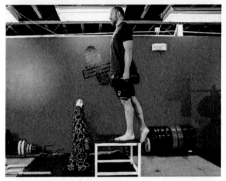

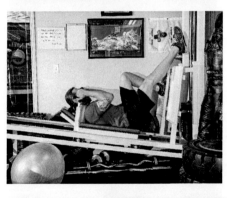

1-leg Press

Use a lying leg press machine, perform the press, but using only one leg. To avoid excess stress on the knee, keep your foot up high and drive through your heel, just like on the step-up. Stay stable, not allowing your knee to travel laterally at all. Perform the movement slow and in a controlled manner until you are confident of your stability. Then if you want to increase the speed of the concentric (pushing) phase of the movement, that is fine, but keep the eccentric (lowering) phase of the movement slow.

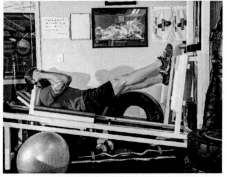

Single Leg Knee Dominant Exercises

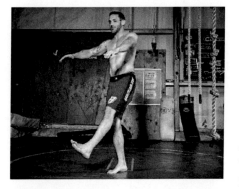

Pistol

The Pistol is a great leg and hip exercise that you can do anywhere and will challenge even the strongest athletes. It is also great for balance and is an exercise you will never be able to di if you don't stabilize your core correctly.

Begin standing on one leg with your arms held out in front of you. Tighten everything from the shoulders down and hold this tension for the entire movement. This will stabilize your lumbar spine, hips, and knees, making it much easier to balance.

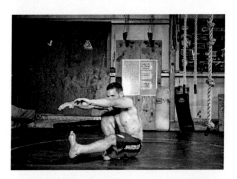

Keep your entire foot flat on the floor with your weight distributed evenly throughout your foot. Slowly sit back, lowering on one le until your cheeks hit the floor. Keep full body tension and reverse the movement to stand up. When you master this, you may start performing the exercise holding a kettlebell in the goblet position, or two kettlebells in the front rack position.

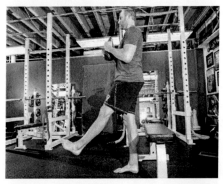

Bench Pistol

If you are struggling with the balance, mobility, or strength to perform a full range of motion pistol, you can also perform the top portion of the movement by lowering to sit on a bench, plyometric box, or heavy bag instead of the floor. As you gain strength, you can gradually sit to lower and lower objects until you can go all the way to the floor.

This is also a good exercise for stronger athletes to overload the top portion of the movement. Even if you can perform the full range of motion pistol, it can be beneficial to mix in partial range bench pistols with a heavy kettlebell.

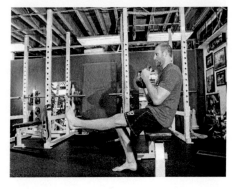

Ninja Jump

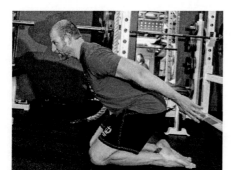

The Ninja Jump (or shin jump), is a good exercise to train rapid extension of the hips and knees followed by rapid flexion to bring the feet back under.

Begin by kneeling on the floor or a mat with your toes pointed behind you. Begin with a quick countermovement, dropping your hips and shoulders down while swinging your arms down and back. Immediately switch directions at the bottom of the countermovement to forcefully extend your hips and knees to drive yourself off of the floor. As soon as your shins and feet clear the floor, quickly pull your knees forward to bring your feet underneath you.

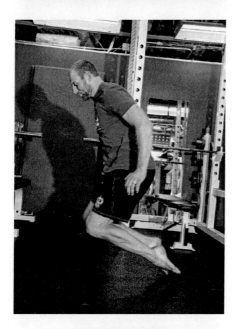

As you begin to master this movement, you can start jumping from your shins onto bumper plates, stacked flooring mats, or small plyometric boxes. Like other box jumps, gradually increase height of your jump over time as you become more proficient at the exercise.

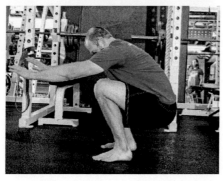

Plyometric Exercises

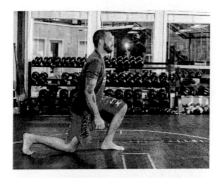

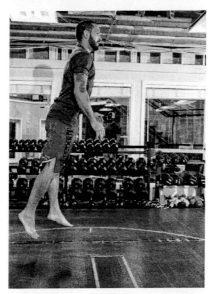

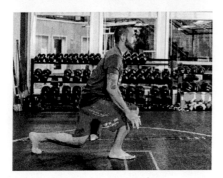

Split Squat Jump

    A good hip dominant exercise to train explosive power from the lunge postition (think takedowns) as well as quick stride turn-over.

    Begin in the lunge postition with back knee just above or gently touching the floor. Though both will contribute, use primarily the front leg to explode out of this position and into the air. Once you clear the floor with full hip extension, quickly switch legs to land in a lunge on the opposite side. Landing in this position also trains your body to stabilize through deceleration which will help to prevent knee injury. Because this movement challenges stability and is explosive in nature, do not perform if you cannot stabilize your knees during it or if your basic lunge technique is sketchy.

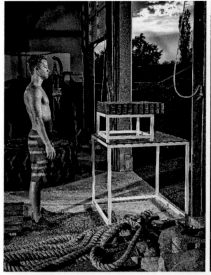
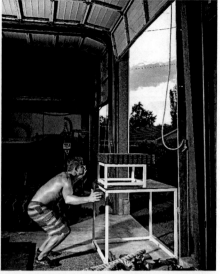
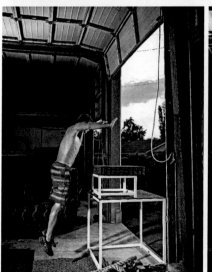
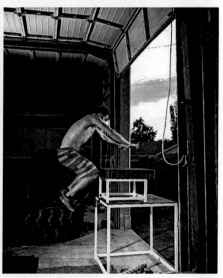
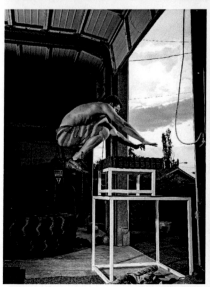
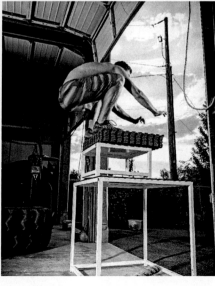

Plyometric Exercises

Box Jump

For the basic box jump, you will stand in front of a plyometric box, make a countermovement and explode off of the floor up onto the box. Start small, and gradually work your way up. Most boxes make 6" jumps from size to size. We will frequently use 1/2" puzzle mats (as shown in photo) to increase height in smaller increments. Your mind will likely give up before your ability to land atop the box, but it is hard to jump well when your confidence wavers. Take it slow, box jump injuries are messy.

A couple of things we will do differently than you may have done in the past.

1) We require that the entire foot lands atop the box, not just the toes or ball of the foot. This makes it much harder to slip and destroy your shins.

2) Never use box jumps for conditioning. We use box jumps as an explosive power exercise, meaning your reps per set will be minimal. This ensures each rep is a focused max effort that will improve your power production and minimize your chance of injury. Most box-jump falls happen during high rep sets while fatigued.

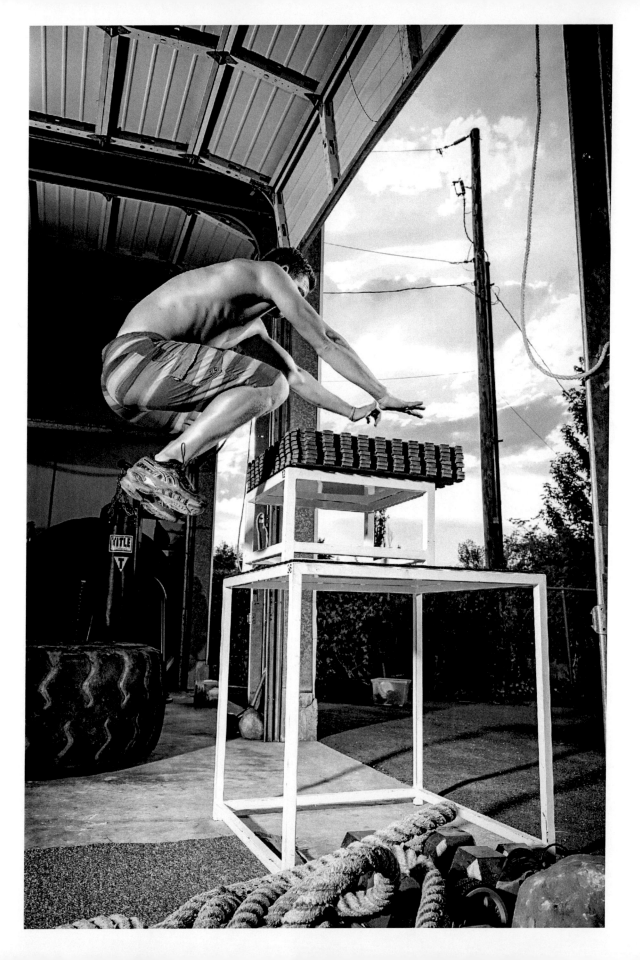

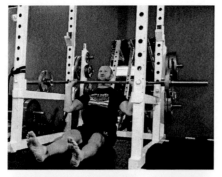

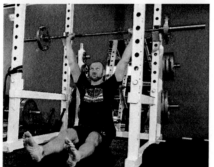

Savickas Press

Named after Lithuanian strongman, Zydrunas Savickas, the Savickas Press is essentially a Military Press while seated on the floor instead of a bench. Straighten your legs out in front of you with the saftey bars of a squat rack set right about shoulder height. In addition to increasing core involvement, this position eliminates your ability to use your legs, making the Savickas a strict press. Begin with the bar on the safety bars. Grasp the bar to lift it off the safety bars, squeeze your shoulder blades together and press the bar overhead without falling over backwards.

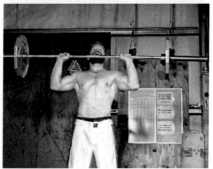

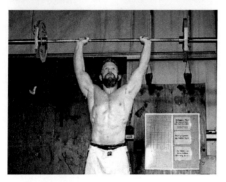

Push Press

The Push Press is a standing shoulder press. You can either start by cleaning the bar to the shoulders, or start with the bar around shoulder height on a squat rack. This lift can either be performed as a strict press with no leg assistance, or with a slight knee bend and bounce, allowing you to press more weight. Either way, squeeze your shoulder blades together and draw your ribs in to stabilize your core as you press the weight overhead and slowly control the decent of the bar to the starting position.

Vertical Push Exercises

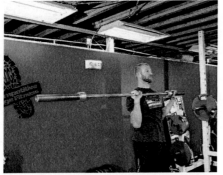

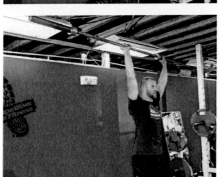

Offset Push Press

This is a great press to really challenge your core. Set up just like a Push Press, but begin with much less weight and one hand in the center of the bar. Slowly press up, attempting to keep the entire bar parallel to the floor for the duration of the movement. You can do half of your repetitions and then switch hand positions for the remaining reps, or if doing an even number of sets, just do one position each set.

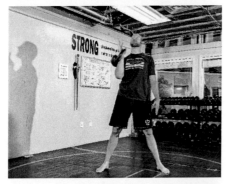

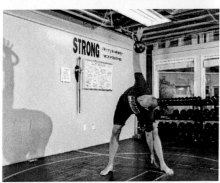

Bent Press (Also a Rotation Exercise)

With your feet wide, hold a dumbbell, kettlebell, or barbell in the front rack position by your shoulder. Hinge at the hips, pushing them back while rotating to press the weight up with one hand and reach toward the floor with the opposite hand. Be sure to lock your lumbar spine in a neutral position, hinging at the hips rather than bending at the waist. Keep the weight directly above your shoulder for the entire movement. It helps to keep your eyes on the weight for the duration of the exercise.

Once you have pressed the weight, reverse the movement to lower the weight while standing back up.

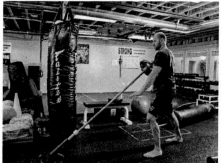

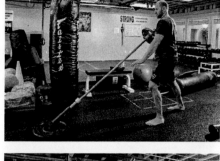

<u>**Landmine Punch Press**</u> **(Also a Rotation Exercise)**

The Landmine Punch Press is a 1-arm Shoulder Press with a slight squat and big rotation. Begin in a staggered stance with your right foot back and the barbell in right hand. Drop your right shoulder back and lower into a slight squat. Explode through into a shoulder press with a big rotation, driving your right hand, shoulder and the barbell forward. Perform this movement as explosively as possible.

WHAT IS A LANDMINE?

The Landmine is a sleeve for the end of a barbell that pivots and rotates in any direction. You can buy a landmine that is attached to a metal base plate, or a landmine like the one in the photo that has a small post that you slide into a bumper plate. Both work great, but the one pictured will save you some money.

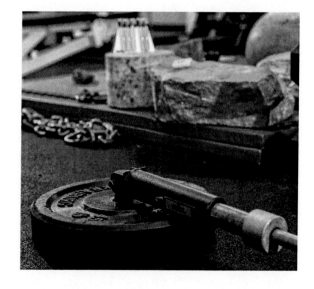

Horizontal Pull Exercises

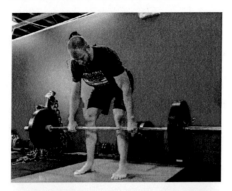

Bent-over Row

In addition to being a horizontal pull, this exercise is essentially a mid-movement isometric dead-lift. Begin by dead-lifting the bar from the floor. From standing, bend the knees slightly while hinging at the hips, driving them back to lower the shoulders. Maintain a neutral spine and squeeze your shoulder blades together as you bring your elbows back to draw the bar to your upper abdomen. Pause and then control the bar back to the bottom position.

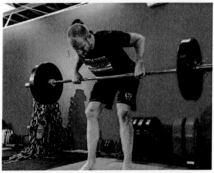

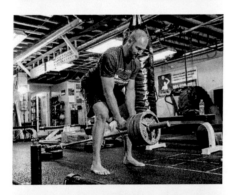

Landmine Row

This is a Bent-over Row using the landmine. Straddle the bar and hinge the hips to grab the bar. Keep the knees slightly bent, hips back and spine neutral. You can use just your hands on the bar, or use a triangle attachment from a cable machine to hold the bar. Perform just as you would a Bent-over Row.

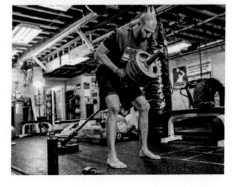

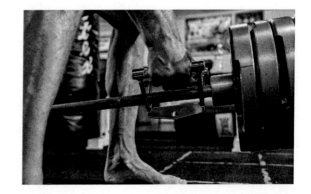

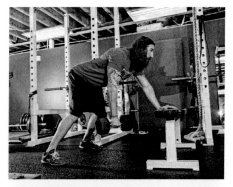

1-arm DB Row

This differs from a standard 1-arm DB Row because you will have both feet back rather than doing the movement with one knee on the bench. Having both feet back requires a little more stability and core involvement.

Place both feet slightly wider than shoulder width apart and bend knees slightly into an athletic stance. Place one hand on the bench while grasping a dumbbell with the other. Squeeze your shoulder blades and bring the dumbbell up beside your upper abdomen. Pause for 1-2 seconds, then return to starting position.

Keep your upper back engaged for the entire movment to not allow your shoulder to rotate forward.

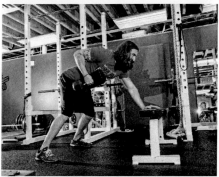

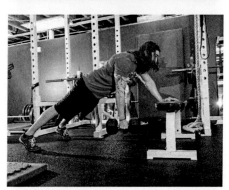

DB Tripod Row

Similar to the 1-arm DB Row, but instead of being in an athletic stance, extend your hips and knees all the way back into a near plank position. The support arm should be roughly perpendicular to the torso and the feet kept wide to minimize hip rotation. Try and keep your hips parallel to the floor, not allowing the right hip to raise as you row the dumbell toward your side. As with the 1-arm DB Row, keep the shoulder blades pinched together and don't allow the shoulder to rotate forward as you perform the movement.

As you likely expect, performing the exercise in a plank position makes it much more core intensive and challenging.

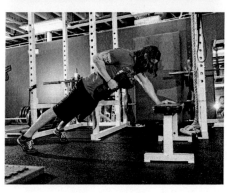

Horizontal Pull Exercises

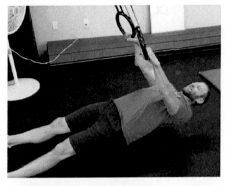

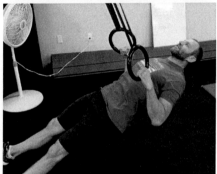

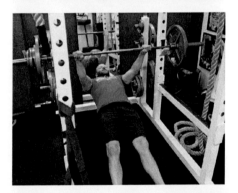

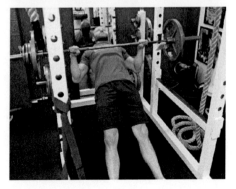

Inverted Row

The inverted Row can be done on rings or on a barbell in a squat rack. The lower the rings or bar, the harder the exercise will be.

Begin suspended from the rings, holding your body in a straight line from shoulders to ankles. Squeeze your shoulder blades together and pull yourself up to the rings. As you lift your body up, use only your upper back, do not lead with your hips to generate momentum. Pause for 1-2 seconds at the top of the movement. As you return to the starting position, do not relax your core to let your hips sag at the bottom of the movement.

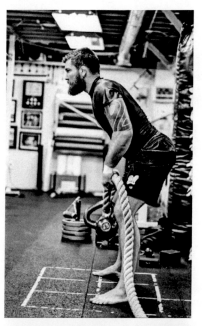

KB Rope Row (Also a Grip Exercise)

The Kettlebell Rope Row is essentially a Bent-over Row, but using a battle rope and kettlebells instead of a bar. Feed your rope through the handles of a kettlebell or kettlebells for desired weight. Straddle the kettlebells and grasp the rope fairly close beside them. Bend the knees slightly and push the hips back while hinging forward. Keep your back straight and squeeze your shoulder blades together during the entire movement.

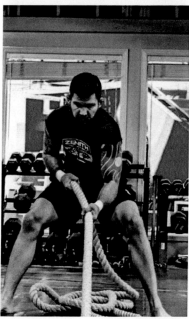

Rope Pull (Also a Grip Exercise)

Begin with a battle rope attached to a 45 lb. weight plate (we use a loop of climbing webbing threaded through a knot in the rope and the handle of the plate, then attached end to end with a carabiner). Once you have attached the weight to to the rope, you can add as much resistance as necessary by piling dumbbells on top of the weight plate. Rubber flooring is ideal for this exercise, but carpet and turf will also work. The weight will slide significantly easier on carpet or turf, so you will have to use more dumbbells.

Once you are set up, stand at the end of the rope, facing the weight plate. Bend your hips and knees slightly to maintain your balance, and begin pulling the weight hand over hand toward you. Once the plate reaches you, walk the rope back to where the plate started and pull it back.

Horizontal Push Exercises

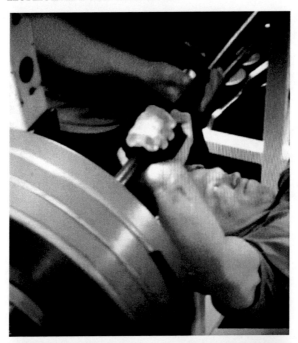

Bench Press

Lay on the bench, grasp the bar and squeeze your shoulder blades together tightly before you lift the bar off of the rack. Keeping your shoulders pinched tight will help to stabilize and protect your shoulders throughout the movement. Once you have lifted the bar off the rack, slowly lower to the center of your chest. Your elbows shouldn't be flared out, or tucked at your sides, rather at approximately 45 degrees. Reverse the movement at the bottom to press the weight back to the starting point. Your hands should be wide enough that as you lower to your chest with elbows about 45 degrees, your hands will be directly above your elbows.

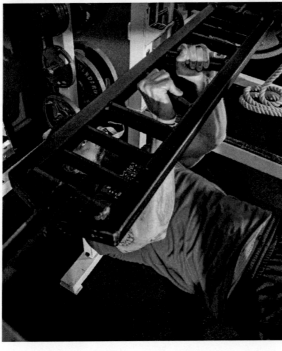

Swiss Bar Bench Press

The Swiss Bar Bench is a variation of the Bench Press which uses a specialty bar to change the angle of the hands. The narrower you hold the handles, the more triceps you use and the wider you get the more it activates the chest. We like a narrow grip, usually using the two most narrow sets of handles as they are more applicable to combat. There is a saying in grappling, "Keep your enemies close and your elbows closer".

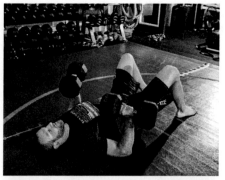

DB Floor Press

The Floor Press is a good alternative to the Bench Press for athletes who are susceptible to shoulder issues. During a bench press, once the elbow breaks 90 degrees, the shoulder extends and internally rotates which presses excessive strain on the glenohumeral joint. If you struggle with shoulder impingement syndrome, this will make it worse. The benefit of the Floor Press is that shoulder extension and internal rotation are eliminated by the floor as it restricts the range of motion of the shoulders.

Perform like a bench press, but lying supine on the floor.

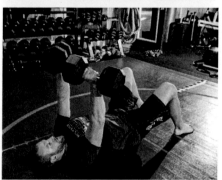

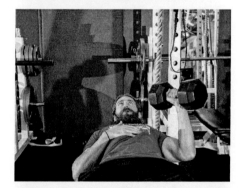

1-arm DB Bench Press

Just like a Bench Press, but with a dumbbell in a single arm. We like the single arm version because it heavily recruits the core to keep you from tipping off the bench as you lower the dumbbell.

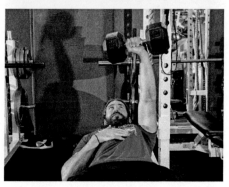

Vertical Pull Exercises

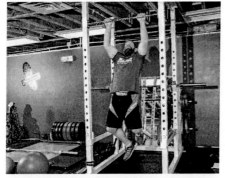

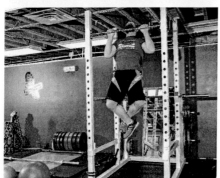

Pull-up

Pull-ups are our favorite vertical pull movement. That being said, they can be hard on many athlete's elbows when done in high volume. This being the case, we like to mix up the grip from workout to workout or even within a single workout. We often rotate between wide and narrow Pull-ups (palms facing away from body), Wide and Narrow Neutral Grip (palms facing each other), Chin-ups (palms facing body) and Archers.

For a basic Pull-up, grasp the bar slightly wider than shoulder width apart. Engage the rhomboids and lats to squeeze your shoulder blades back and down, then pull your elbows to your sides to raise your chin over the bar. Lower back down under control. Pause at near extension without loosing tension and repeat (we also occassionally dead-hang with full elbow extension and relaxation at the bottom, but not everyone's shoulders and elbows will tolerate it).

Some people make the rest of us look bad doing pull-ups, so we happily allow them to use external resistance such as chains, dumbbells, and weight vests. If you are unable to do pull-ups, start with negatives.

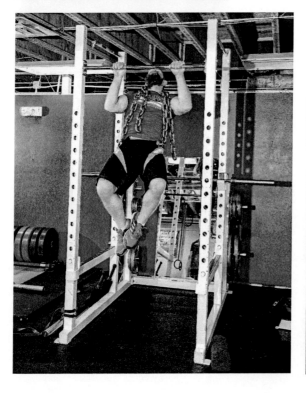

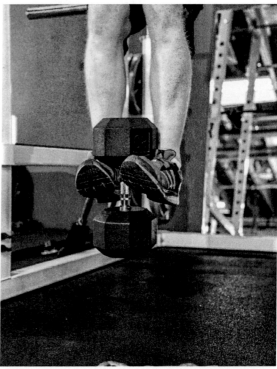

Vertical Pull Exercises

Treadmill Plank Pull

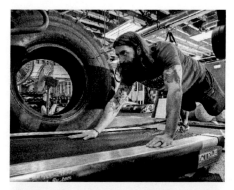

Make sure the treadmill is turned off. Place one hand on the side of the treadmill, then reach with the other hand to put your palm flat on the belt. Press down on the belt and pull with your lats and abs to move the belt. Do half of your repetitions on one side, then switch hands and repeat.

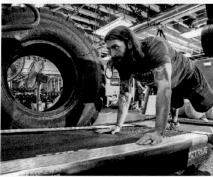

Mixed Grip Chin-up

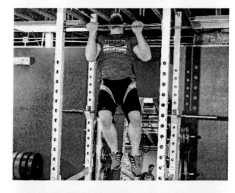

Similar to a mixed grip on the a Dead-lift, mixing your grip on a Chin-up makes it easier to hold on to the bar. This makes it slightly easier than a regular Chin-up, but also increases core engagement to keep your body from rotating. Switch hand position half way through your repetitions, or from set to set.

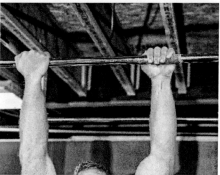

Vertical Pull Exercises

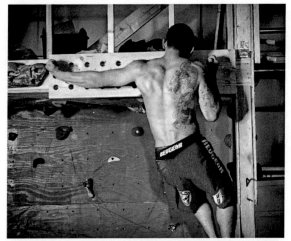

Archer

This is an extremely difficult exercise that requires stabilization of the spine while the athlete is moving slowly through a highly demanding upper body movement. This can be done on a peg board as pictured, or on a pull-up bar.

Begin by pulling yourself up to a point where your chin is just above the bar. While keeping yourself at the same height, slowly pull yourself over to one hand. Pause, then slowly pull your body toward the other hand.

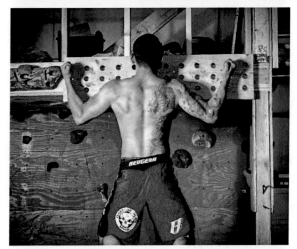

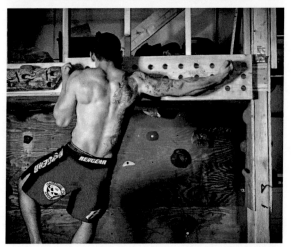

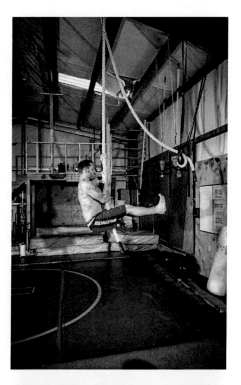

Rope Climb

Rope climbing is an awesome vertical pull movement. If you haven't climbed ropes before, definitely start with using your feet. Holding yourself up with your hands, bring your right foot underneath the rope from the left side so the rope is laying across your right foot. Bring your left foot across the top of the rope to pinch the rope between your feet. You should essentially be able to stand up on your left foot, with the rope trapped between your feet.

If this is going well, try to climb (even if you just go up and down the bottom portion of the rope) the rope using only your upper body. Initially, pull with both arms simultaneously, using that momentum to move the bottom hand up. As you get stronger, try only to pull with the top hand as the bottom hand reaches to grab further up on the rope.

Lastly, if you are able, hold your legs out in front of you while using only your arms like Lucus is doing in the photos.

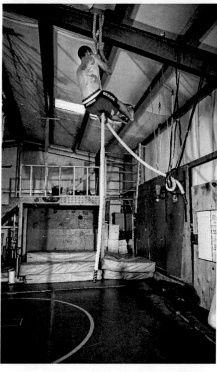

Vertical Pull Exercises

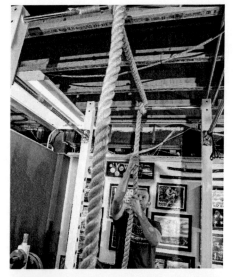

Rope Climber

Not every gym will have a rope to climb. While not the same, a decent alternative is to wrap a battle rope around the cross braces of a squat rack. One complete loop around each cross brace is a good place to start. Make sure the loops are going the same direction, or the rope will get bound up.

Once the rope is set up, begin on the short side and pull the rope hand over hand until you have pulled the majority of the rope to you. Go to the other side and repeat. This can be done standing, kneeling, or seated. It is easier to cheat standing up, by dropping your hips to use your bodyweight to pull, not just your arms. Sitting eliminates this possibility. If it is too easy, add another loop on one side or have your battle buddy add just a little bit of friction with their hand on the rope.

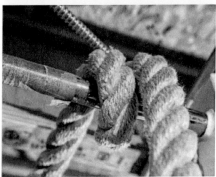

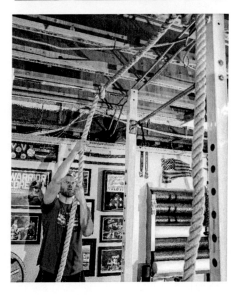

Rotation/Anti-Rotation Exercises

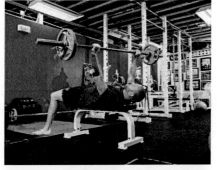

G Twist

Start the exercise as you would a bench press, lying on a bench with hands grasping a barbell slightly wider than shoulder width apart. Put your feet out wide to prevent yourself from falling off the bench. Keeping your arms relatively straight, lower one side of the bar to touch the floor without letting your shoulder blades come off the bench. Keep your back pressed firmly against the bench and reach with your arms rather than letting your torso twist. Once you tap the end of the bar to the floor, simultaneously brace your abs, pull up and across your body with the arm that is up and raise the arm that is down in a chest fly motion. Begin with just the 45 lb. bar, and add weight as needed.

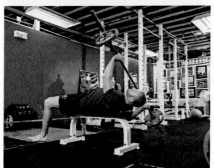

Hanging Windshield Wiper

The Hanging Windshield Wiper is a very challenging rotation exercise where you must pull your hips and legs up in front of you, then hold them there while you rotate your hips from side to side.

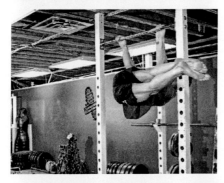

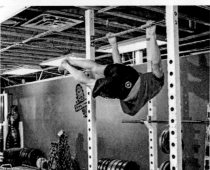

Rotation/Anti-Rotation Exercises

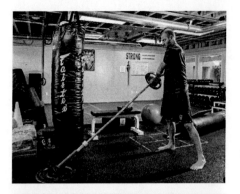

Landmine Rotation

Start the exercise facing the landmine with your feet shoulder width apart. Grasp the end of the bar with both hands above and in front of your head. Keep your elbows as straight as possible while slowly rotating your shoulders from side to side. Keep your hips pointed at the landmine and only rotate as far as you can without rotating your hips. Brace your core and don't allow your lumbar spine to arch during the movement.

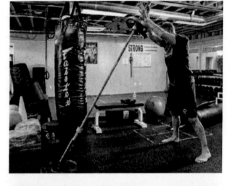

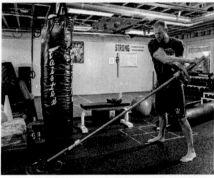

Rotation/Anti-Rotation Exercises

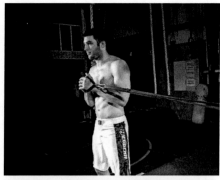

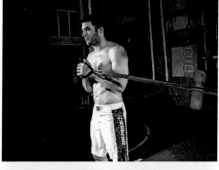

Pallof Press

Stand perpendicular to a superband (1/2" band for endurance or 1" band for strength) or cable machine with your feet slightly wider than shoulder width apart. With the band or cable in your hands at the center of your chest, brace your core, and slowly extend your arms in a straight line. The resistance will try to pull your hands away from the centerline as you extend your arms. Don't let it. The further you extend and the slower you go, the more challenging this exercise will be. Each repetition should take at least 10 seconds. As a general rule - when you think you are doing the exercise right - go slower.

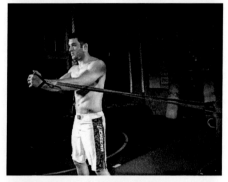

Waterball Lunge Twist (Also a Hip Dominant Exercise)

Begin by hugging a waterball (instructions on page) to your chest. Step forward into a lunge, then rotate over the front knee with the ball. Focus on keeping the front knee directly over the foot and not allowing it to drift laterally with the rotation. Return to center and step into the next lunge with the opposite foot.

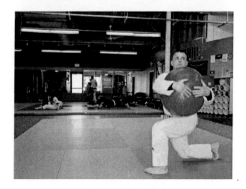

Rotation/Anti-Rotation Exercises

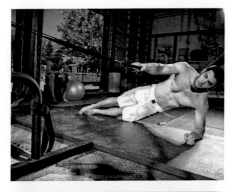

Side Plank Pull

Start in a side plank position facing either a cable machine or a superband (1" band is a good place to start). While keeping your spine in a straight line from cranium to sacrum, squeeze your shoulder blades together to slowly pull the band or cable towards you. Pause 1-2 seconds before returning to the starting position with the top arm extended in front of you. Try not to let your hips dip below the centerline of your body.

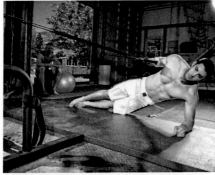

Side Plank Press

Begin in the same plank position as the Side Plank Pull, but facing away from the band. Grab the band over your top arm and hold the band near your chest. Again, do not let your hips dip below the centerline of your body.

Squeeze your shoulder blades to stabilize the movement and slowly push the band in front of you. Pause 1-2 seconds before returning to the starting postition.This is quite a bit harder than the Side Plank Pull and keeping your balance is very challenging.

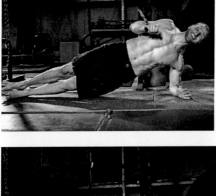

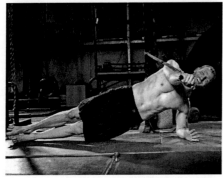

Plyometric Exercises

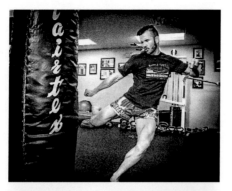

Heavy Bag Kicks

Kicking a heavy bag is a great, explosive rotational exercise. If you are an MMA fighter, you will likely get plenty of this in your striking workouts, however, you may also consider pairing this with a heavy rotational strength exercise (G-Twist, Landmine Rotation, Hanging Windshield Wiper, etc.) during complex training. Play around with both low and high kicks as they will each challenge your core differently.

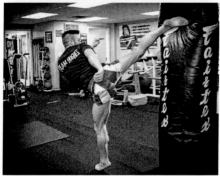

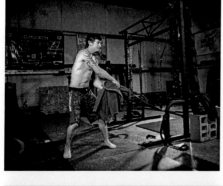

Reverse Superband Chop

The Reverse Superband Chop is a great way to train explosive rotation from a low level to a high level. Begin perpendicular to a superband attached at or near floor level. You can attach a handle to the band, or slip a gi top or gi pants through the bend. This is a great way to work on dynamic grip strength while performing the rotational exercise. Start in a partial squat position, bent over at the waist, but with back straight and shoulders rotated toward the band attachment. Explosively stand and rotate the opposite direction to bring the gi or handle from beside your left knee to above your right shoulder. Do the movement only as powerfully as you can while maintaining control.

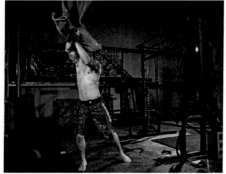

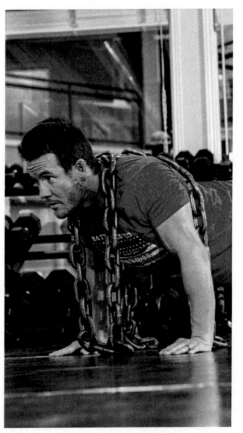

Chapter 10
Test Specific

Chapter 10 - Test Specific

Mililtary branches and law enforcement agencies have fitness tests that some of you may need to prepare for. As this book is directed toward people who are likely already very physically fit you can probably already pass your PT test with flying colors. Great. Our goal is for you to dominate the test and score among the very top performers. In specialty programs everyone can meet the standard, but as the SEALs say, "It pays to be a winner."

Most PT tests consist at minimum of push-ups, sit-ups, and a 1.5-2 mile run, so those are the exercises we will focus on. The obvious way is to improve muscular endurance to do more repetitions. Another often neglected approach is to improve strength in the movement we are testing. The stronger I am, the easier each repetition will be and the more capable I will be of performing more repetitions. By training both methods we will improve both strength and endurance, taking your PT score to superior levels.

In this chapter, you will find exercises and methods both to increase your number of repetitions as well as what we term "resisted" movements that will help you increase your strength in the specific movement (for example, the chain push-up pictured on the previous page). Some of these movements will be included in other parts of the program. If you need to raise your PT score, follow the instructions below.

I do not believe that a test made up of push-ups, sit-ups, and a run is a very good indicator of overall fitness or of a persons ability to perform the physical tasks his career might demand. Too often we see soldiers and police officers who train simply to pass the PT test and neglect full body, functional fitness. Agility, strength, intermittent sprinting, and ability to carry load, are all better indicators of a tactical athletes fitness and ability to perform in the field. In addition, a program that emphasizes push-ups and sit-ups can lead to other problems. This being the case, once you can dominate the requirements of the PT test, our Test Specific training will enter a maintenance phase and much more importance will be placed on the Task Specific training methods found in the following chapter.

I Need To Improve My Score

If you are preparing for a PT test, you will train each movement at least twice a week. You can add these to the workouts, subbing out Task Specific portions, or just doing it all. One time a week will be a high repetition day and the other will be a resisted day to build strength.To make it personal, set a goal for push-ups and sit-ups. Here is what to do:

On Strength Days - Your total number of reps should equal your goal. Break it into as many sets as necessary and gradually get it done in fewer sets.
On Endurance Days - Do one consecutive set of your goal reps. Repeat for at least half of your goal on the second set.

TSAC Test Specific - Resisted Push-ups

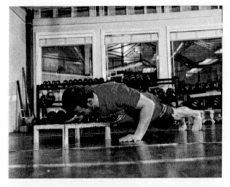

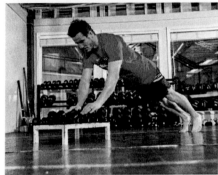

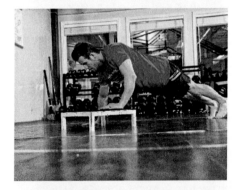

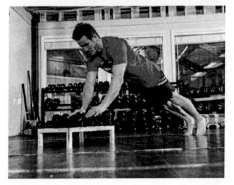

Box Cross Push-up

The Box Cross Push-up is a resisted push-up. By doing push-ups with your hands at different heights, you get more range of motion on the shoulder complex of the top hand. Also, once you near the top of the push-up, the shoulder complex of the bottom hand can no longer assist in the movement, overloading this side.

Begin with one hand on a 6" plyometric box or medicine ball. Do a push-up, then explosively cross over to land with the opposite hand on the box or medicine ball. Keep crossing back and forth as explosively as possible for desired number of reps.

TSAC Test Specific - Resisted Push-up

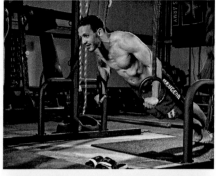

Ring Push-up

The Ring Push-up is a resisted push-up that challenges the stability of the exercise during the movement. Placing your hands on the rings greatly increases core engagement, requiring full body tension just to hold the position.

Start with the rings approximately one foot above the floor. Place your hands on the rings in a push-up postition, squeezing your shoulder blades together and holding your core tight to avoid letting your lower back sag. While maintaining core tension, slowly lower into the bottom of push-up. Pause and slowly reverse the movement to return to the starting position. The lower the rings, the more difficult the exercise will be.

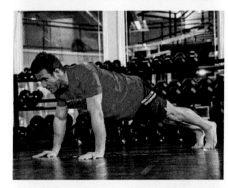

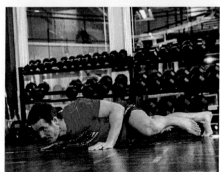

Spiderman Push-up

The Spiderman Push-up increases load on the chest, shoulders and triceps by bringing more of your bodyweight toward the front of your body. As you lower down, lean to one side and bring the opposite knee up toward your elbow.

TSAC Test Specific - Resisted Push-up

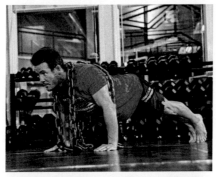

Chain Push-up

Push-ups can also be easily loaded with chains, weight vests or bands to make them more challenging and to build more strength in the push-up movement.

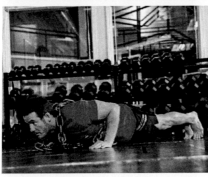

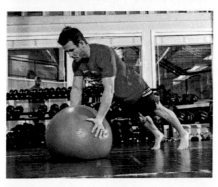

Stability Ball Push-up

Performing push-ups on a stability ball is more challenging due to the instability of the ball. This causes neural recruitment of more muscle fibers which will carry over when you go back to normal push-ups.

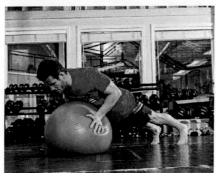

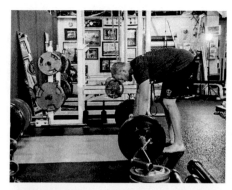

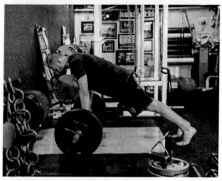

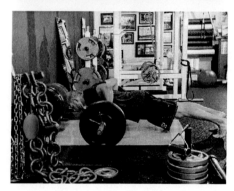

TSAC Test Specific - Resisted Push-up

Barbell Roll-out to Push-up

Another challenging unstable push-up is the Barbell Roll-out to Push-up. Start with a barbell on the floor with anywhere from 10-45 lb. plates. Stand with your shins next to the bar and put your hands on the bar directly below your shoulders. Roll the bar forward and lower your hips into a push-up position. Perform 1-2 push-ups, then pull with your feet to bring the barbell back to your shins.

TSAC Test Specific - Push-up Endurance

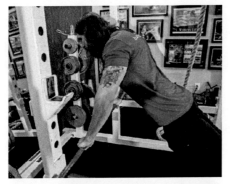

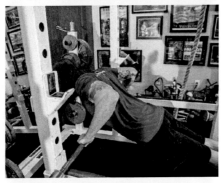

Bar Push-up

The easiest way to do more push-ups is to make them easier. This is a great way to improve endurance. By elevating your hands, you can adjust the push-up to reach your PT test goal. If your goal is 80 push-ups, set the bar on a squat rack at a height that you can do 80 straight push-ups. When you have done 80 push-ups at that height, lower the bar for the next endurance workout and do it again. Keep lowering the bar gradually over time until you can do 80 on the floor.

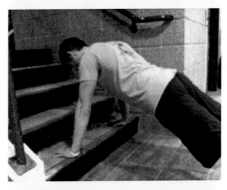

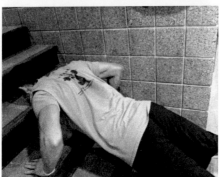

Stair Push-up

An alternative to the Bar Push-up is the Stair Push-up. Following the same concept, start high and gradually work your way down. An alternative is to do as many push-ups as you can on the floor, then immediately to the first stair for a few more. Each time you fatigue, move up one stair to make the push-ups a little easier in effort to get a few more repetitions.

TSAC Test Specific - Push-up Endurance

Reverse Grip Bar Push-up

Another spin on the elevated push-up is to perform Reverse Grip Bar Push-ups. Basically you just reverse your hands to an underhand grip, scoot your hands in to just wider than hip width apart and do high repetition push-ups. This really burns out the triceps.

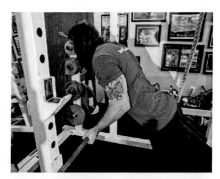

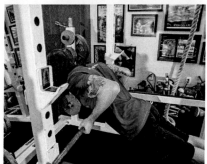

2-Minute Plank

If you are taking a 2-minute PT test, you need to make sure you can hold a plank for at least 2 minutes. If not, regardless of your upper body endurance, your core will give out before you are done. Start planking.

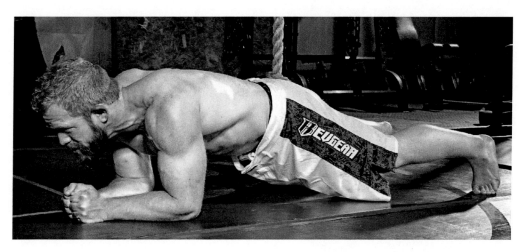

TSAC Test Specific - Sit-up Strength

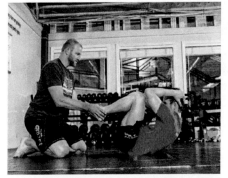

Tuck and Roll

The Tuck and Roll exercise is a partner assisted exercise. One partner assumes a sit-up position, but places his elbows on his knees. This partner's number 1 goal is to keep his elbows directly on his knees, not allowing any space between elbows and knees and not allowing his elbows to slide down his legs.

The second partner kneels in front of the other's feet, grabs his ankles, and proceeds to roll his partner back and forth, up and down and side to side. Go until the partner being rolled gives up. You will be amazed at how hard this is.

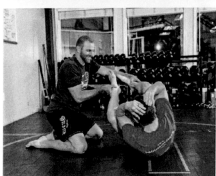

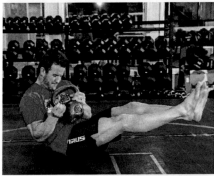

Kettlebell Russian Twist

For the Russian Twist, hold a kettlebell by the sides, lean back slightly, and lift your feet off the ground. Slowly rotate your shoulders to move the kettlebell from side to side.

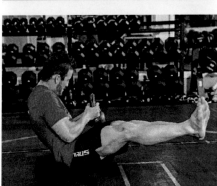

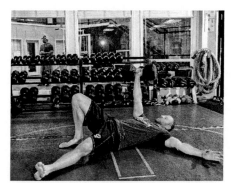

The Half Get-up

The Half Turkish Get-up is a great exercise to strengthen your core. The full Get-up is also obviously great for the core, but the weight you are able to use is limited both by mobility and by leg strength. By only performing a Half Get-up, you are increasing your ability to add weight because it is only a partial movement, mimicking the Sit-up more closely and placing your abdominal muscles in more constant time-under-tension.

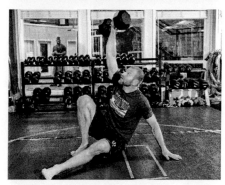

You can use a kettlebell, dumbbell, or a heavy bag over the shoulder. I lean toward the heavy bag for test specific Sit-Up training, but any of the options are great.

Perform just like the first portion of the Turkish Get-up. Start with the weight in one arm (or on one shoulder) and the knee on that side up. Shift your hips out to that side. Use your opposite arm and core to raise up to a seated position. Reverse the movement to return to start.

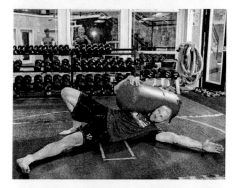

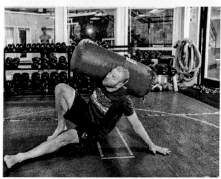

TSAC Test Specific - Sit-up Endurance

The Combat Sit-up

    I'm not a huge fan of sit-ups as repeated lumbar flexion is not great for spines over time. I AM a huge fan of grappling though, so when someone has to do sit-ups for a PT test, we encourage them to try these. We have found the number of combat sit-ups an athlete can do in a given time correlates fairly well with the number of sit-ups they can do. Essentially, you will start on your back with a partner in your guard and sit up to the side as if doing a hip-bump sweep. This is a great movement that leads to the sweep, a kimura and a guillotine. A sit-up that is also practical is something I can support!

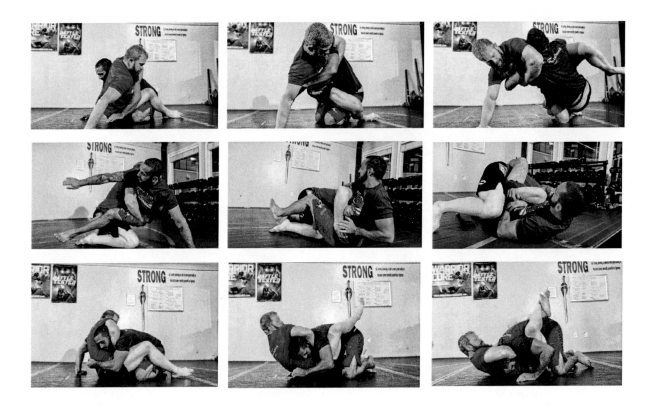

Paddleboat

The Paddleboat can be used to improve endurance or strength, depending how heavy of weight if any you decide to hold. You will sit down, hold your arms above your chest (with or without weight), lean back slightly, and begin to flex and extend your hips and knees. Obviously, the heavier the weight you use, the harder the exercise. Holding weight only in one hand will also make it more challenging as it increases the difficulty of balancing.

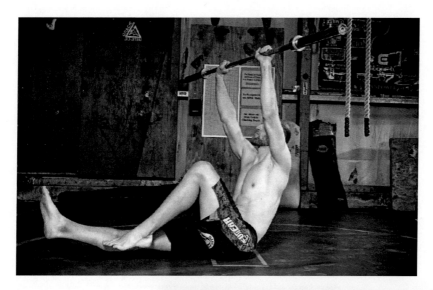

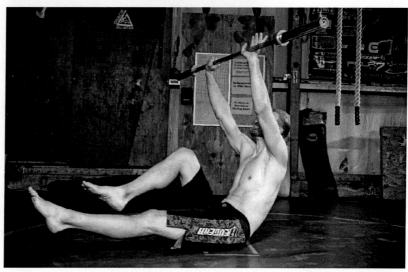

TSAC Test Specific - Sit-up Endurance

Banded Dead Bug

The Banded Dead Bug is also good for training endurance, though you likely won't be able to hold it very long initially. Begin like you would the Dead Bug in the correctives section, however, hold your arms directly above your chest, while holding tension on a 1/2" superband pulling from behind you. Keep your lumbar spine glued to the floor and your shoulder blades up, just off of the floor. Hold for as long as possible, then switch sides.

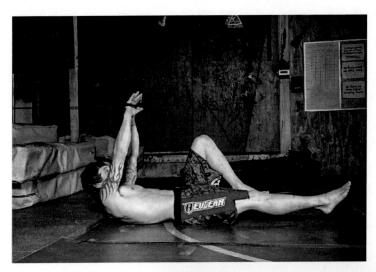

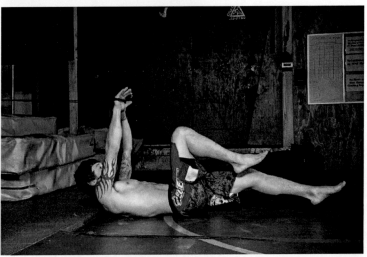

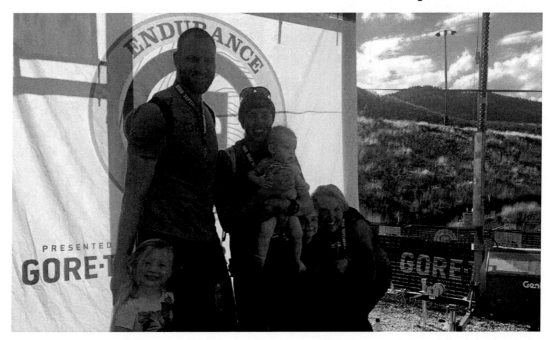

Nutshell Running

A few years ago, we started making shirts that say "I Run." To date, I get more comments from strangers about that shirt than from the entire rest of my wardrobe combined. Just yesterday, I wore one for the first time in months while making my monthly Costco trip. Sure enough, two ladies stopped me within minutes to question me about my shirt. For some reason, people seem bonded, or connected by running. I always feel slightly guilty, but not without an genuine smile as I turn to reveal the lifter overhead squatting on the back of the shirts right below the words, "...as little as possible."

Running has never been my thing. It's ironic then that my wife is an ultra-marathoner. One of my biggest issues with running is that most people who run, run too much and neglect everything else. Over-training/under-recovery is a huge problem with many aspiring runners. When my wife ran her first 50-miler, the longest race she had done was a half marathon. She trained for 3 months, running only 2-3 times a week,. We emphasized recovery (only 1 long run/week and a fair amount of bodywork) and she made it through the training and race without any over-use injuries.

I tell that story simply to prove a point that you don't need to run 4-5 days a week to get better at running! I ran the above pictured North Face Endurance Challenge 50K on a couple months of training 1-2 days a week. I ran 27 miles once with my wife. Beyond that, my longest run was 13 miles. If you are planning to pursue special operations however, you need to run everyday. If not, and you are simply trying to prepare fore a PT test, or to keep your cardio up, 2-3 days a week and emphasizing recovery will likely yield better results and help you avoid plantar fasciitis, shin splints, IT band syndrome, knee pain, hip pain, and low back pain. Plus, it will leave you some time to lift!

Unless you NEED to prepare for intense daily running, try the following 2-3 training days.

TSAC Test Specific - The Run

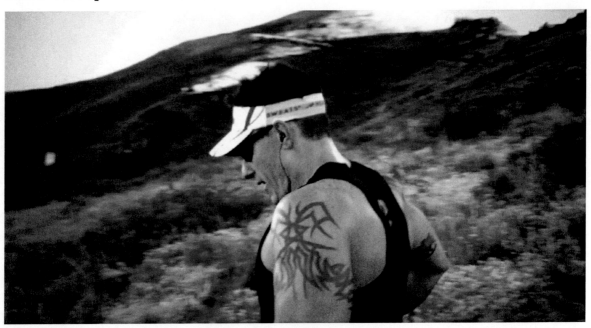

Timed Run

Some PT tests are 1.5 miles, some are 2 miles. Whichever distance your test is, that is the distance you will run. Time yourself initially to see where you are at. Once a week you perform a timed 1.5-2 mile with the goal being to improve every time, working closer and closer to your goal.

Speed Run

It is difficult to get faster if you don't push the pace a little bit. Every second run of your week will be a speed day. Continually alternate between these workouts every speed workout.

8 x 400 meters @ goal pace - 15 seconds
Run as far as possible @ goal pace, when you slow down, stop, rest 2 minutes and repeat.
4 x 800 meters @ goal pace
Hill sprints - Sprint up, jog down, rest 1 minute. 3 @ 75-90% max speed, 12 @ max speed

Goal pace means the speed you need to run to meet your goal. For example, if you want to run a 6-minute mile, your 400 meter laps will be 1:30 and your 800 meter laps will be 3 minutes.

Resisted Run

If you run a third day in a week, make it a resisted day. This means running hills, running with a weight vest or a ruck, or both. Make your run harder than your test will be so that when you get back to flat ground it will seem easy!

Chapter 11
Task Specific

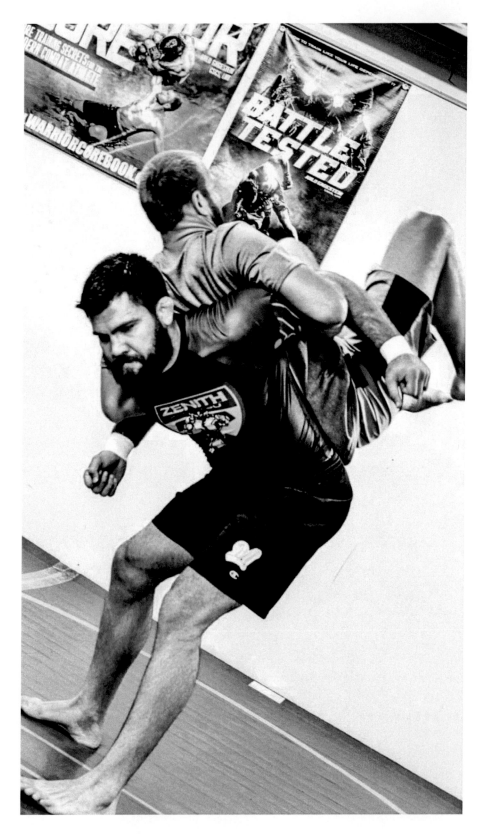

Chapter 11 - Task Specific

As previously mentioned, I don't believe the standard PT test is a great indicator of a tactical athlete's fitness. Nor would push-ups, sit-ups, and a 2-mile run be a good indicator of a fighter's fitness. Depending just on those exercises would leave both individuals very vulnerable when they step into the cage or onto the streets. That is where the Task Specific section of the Battle Tested program comes into play. Where Test Specific prepares you to pass a harmless, unfunctional test, Task Specific prepares you to survive.

On the following pages, you will see drills and circuits that relate in some way to the actual duties of the tactical athlete and the fighter. Some drills will focus on combining ground fighting with strength training movements, others will focus on speed and agility, some will focus on load carriage, and still other drills will mimic the movements and metabolic demands of the combat athlete.

Task Specific Workout 1 - Partner Exercises

<u>TSW 1</u> *Lift-Jitsu non-stop for 20 minutes*

<u>Lift-Jitsu</u>

Lift-Jitsu is the combination of jiu-jitsu sparring and other exercises. If there are two partners, roll a 6-minute round, then both partners stop and perform the other exercises before returning to the mat. In a group of 3, two partners will roll for 3 minutes while the third partner does the exercises. After 3 minutes, partner one leaves the mat to do the exercises while the partner two stays to roll with partner three. Rotating through these three positions, each partner will be on the mat for 2 rounds, then perform the exercises for one round. Almost any exercise can be used, but try to keep them complex, multi-joint movements.

Sparring x 6 minutes (1 or two rounds, depending on number of partners)
Squat Jump x 5 repetitions
Pull-up x 5 repetitions
Heavy Bag Turkish Get-up x 10 repetitions

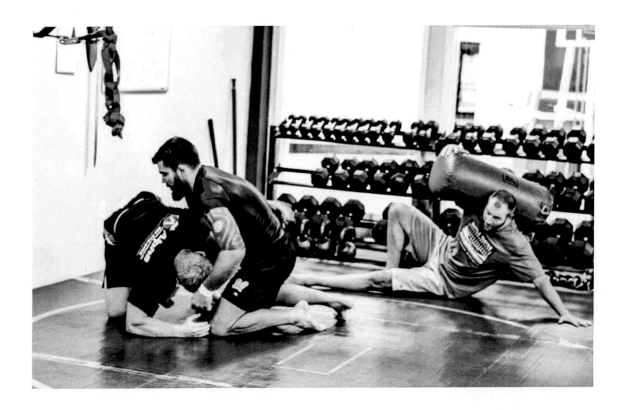

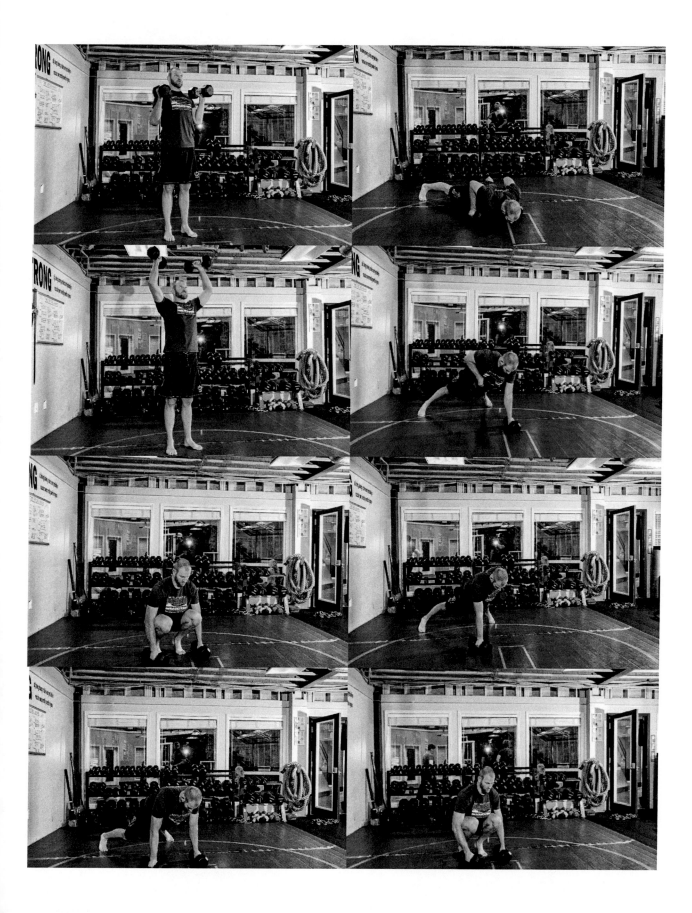

TSW 2

Perform Man Makers for 50 repetitions. This will not be fun.

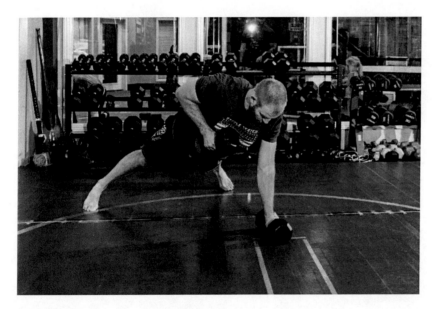

Man Maker

    The Man Maker is essentially a burpee on steroids. Begin with a dumbbell shoulder press, squat down to place the dumbbells on the ground, jump your feet back into a push-up position and perform a push-up. Following the push-up, perform a row with each arm, attempting to keep your hips as parallel to the floor as possible. When the rows are complete, jump your feet back to your hands and return to standing. That is one repetition.

TSW 3

***Carry 1 kettlebell in the rack
position for 1 mile, switching
hands when necessary.***

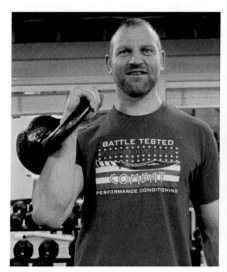 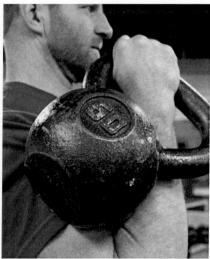

*By holding the kettlebell near the thumb-side bend, you
offset the kettlebell so it won't smash your forearm and
wrist the entire time.*

1-arm Kettlebell Mile

Hold a kettlebell in one hand in the rack position. Engage your core, drawing in your
ribs and bracing your abs as if you are about to be punched. Maintaining this stability,
begin walking. Switch arms as necessary, but continue walking for an entire mile.

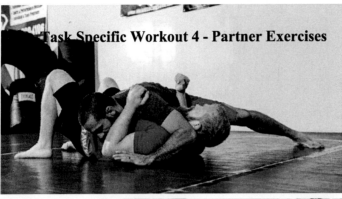

TSW 4

Both partners do all four positions.

Position Drills

Partner 1 attempts to hold Partner 2 in a dominant position for one minute, then rests for 30 seconds. If he is successful, Partner 2 has to complete one of the following:

5 pull-ups
10 squat jumps
15 push-ups
20 bodyweight squats

While none of these are challenging by themselves, they quickly become difficult when they take up the only rest you get between rounds. If Partner 2 escapes within the minute, Partner 1 does the exercise.

You can have one partner start in all four dominant positions (side control, mount, back, north/south) and then switch, or partners can switch controller/escaper, each round

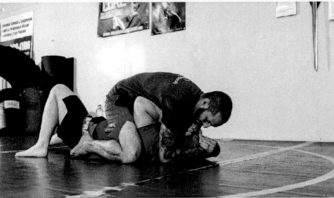

MMA:

Do one minute on, 30 seconds off until both partners have done all four positions. This will take 12 minutes and amount roughly to two pro MMA rounds (including between round rest).

TSAC:

This is a great drill as explained, but you can make it even more applicable with both partners performing a 40yd (or 10 second treadmill) sprint immediately prior to assuming control position. If doing this, feel free to take 60-90 seconds rest between rounds.

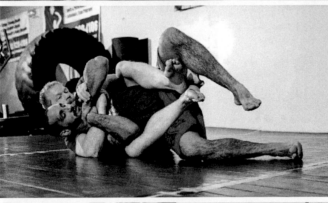

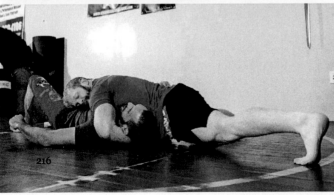

TSW 5

Push-up	***15 sets of 10 repetitions***
Kettlebell Swing	***15 sets of 10 repetitions***
Rope Slam	***15 sets of 10 repetitions***

Perform these exercises as a circuit of 10 reps each. With as little rest as possible, continue to power through 15 sets (150 total reps) of each exercise as fast as possible while maintaining good form.

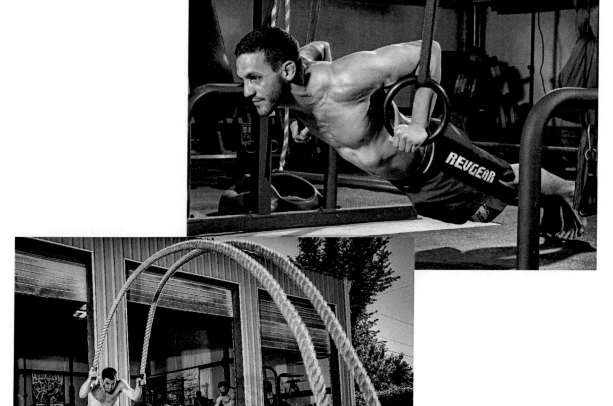

Task Specific Workout 6 - Load Carriage

<u>TSW 6</u> *Perform the Farmer Flip Race for 3-4 Rounds*

<u>Farmer Flip</u>

Alternate a heavy Farmer Carry for 50 yds, followed immediately by a Tire Flip for 50 yds. We use custom made handles to carry the same tire we flip, but you can use any implement (dumbbells, hex bar, strongman axles, etc.) for your carry. This drill is done for speed, but definitely emphasize tall posture and correct technique for both the carries and the flips. This drill is more fun as a competition. Go head to head with a partner or individually time each person in a group. Rest several minutes between rounds.

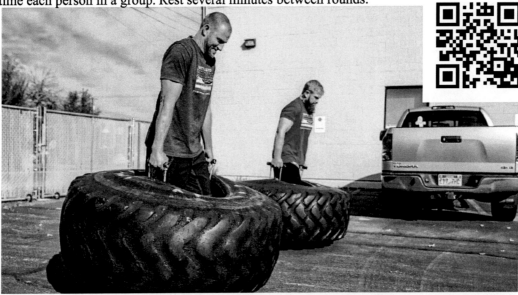

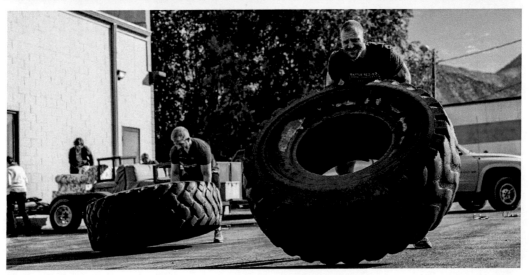

TSW 7

Perform 2 rounds each partner of the Partner Get-up and then 4-5 rounds each partner of the Partner Command Ground and Pound.

Partner Get-up

This is a challenging drill for both partners. As Partner 1 gets from his knees to feet, the Partner 2 needs to maintain his position on the back without hooks or seatbelt position, requiring constant squeeze grip.

With Partner 1 in turtle position, Partner 2 will climb on his back with double underhooks and squeezing the Partner 1's hips with his knees.

Partner 1 will then begin to get to his feet in any way possible. Once Partner 1 is standing, he will reverse the movement to return to his hands and knees.

MMA and TSAC:

Begin with as many get-ups as possible in 2 minutes. As it becomes easier, increase time or find a heavier partner. Rest as necessary, but do 2 rounds each partner.

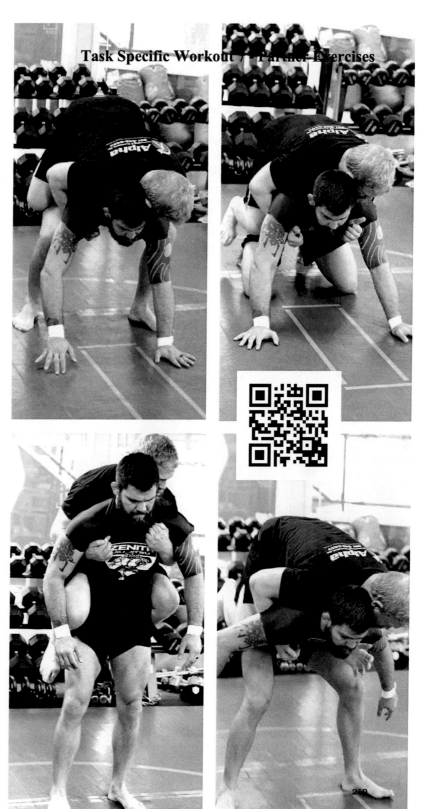

Task Specific Workout 7 - Partner Exercises

Partner Command Ground and Pound

Having a partner shout commands at you while you are ground and pounding makes the drill a little more chaotic as you are never quite sure what to expect. It also trains you to react immediately to instructions from a coach or team leader. This can also take you out of the comfort zone of the positions you always go to and the strikes you always throw.

Partner 1 will start in any position you want on a large heavy bag. When the time starts, he will go all out, 100%, listening to whatever commands Partner 2 gives him. In the following photos, you'll see Lucus commanding the Ginja Ninja, "Strikes! Side cross! Knee on belly! Elbows!" Your partner can command any combination of positions (mount, knee on belly, side control, north/south) and strikes (strikes, hammer fists, elbows, knees).

MMA and TSAC:

Do this drill in 30 second bouts with 90 seconds rest to start. If you are not tired after 30 seconds, you need to strike harder and transition more! As the drill gets easier, increase time to 45, then 60 seconds. Do 4-5 rounds. Decreasing the rest interval will also make it harder.

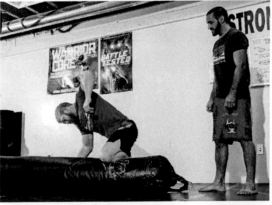
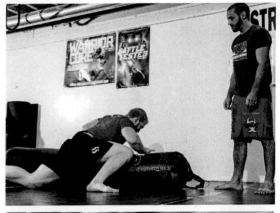
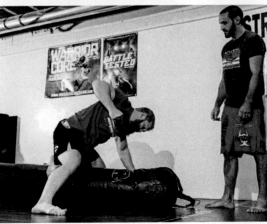
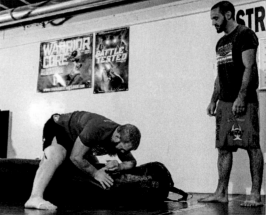

Task Specific Workout 8 - Metabolic Conditioning

TSW 8 *Non-stop Dumbbell Destruction for 10 minutes*

<u>Dumbbell Destruction</u>

Grab two dumbbells. For 10 minutes, do whatever exercises you can think of without stopping. Any dumbbell exercise is fair game. Squats, RDLs, Burpees, Squat Thrusts, Turkish Get-ups, Bent-over Rows, Renegade Rows, Floor Presses, Push Presses, Savickas Presses, Biceps Curls, Pull-overs, Russian Twists, Tricep Extensions, Snatches, Clean and Jerks, etc. The only rule is that you may not rest for 10 minutes.

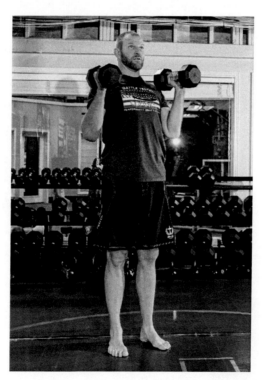

Task Specific Workout 9 - Load Carriage

TSW 9 *Go through the Odd Object Ladder for 4-5 rounds*

The Odd Object Ladder

Similar to an old school ladder on a basketball court, the Odd Object Ladder is a great metabolic drill designed to simulate the physical demands on a tactical athlete. It requires quick, multidirectional movement under load while challenging strength, muscular endurance, and anaerobic capacity. It is very simple to set up with only a park or parking lot and various heavy and/or awkward objects. We typically perform the event as a timed competition between athletes.

Begin by placing 4-5 markers (cones, cinderblocks, etc.) in a line 10 yards apart. At one end, place a heavy object for every marker. We have used dumbbells, sandbags, heavy bags, boulders, bystanders, even old TVs and computer monitors. The participant grabs an item and runs it to the first marker and sprints back for another. One by one, the participant brings an object to each marker, and then starts over to retrieve the objects. The drill is timed. If competing against others, make sure the objects are delivered to markers in the same order.

We really love this drill because it not only mimics a potential military or law enforcement scenario, but it also is extremely adaptable to the capabilities of the trainees. Markers can be added, subtracted, moved further apart, and objects changed, delivery order (for example, heaviest object to furthest marker instead of closest) changed, wearing or not wearing body armor, to account for abilities and progressive overload. This can also be tailored to fire fighters by using stairs.

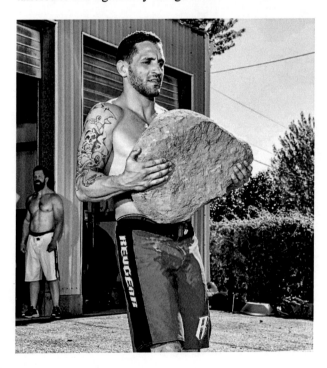

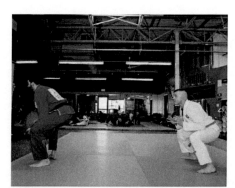

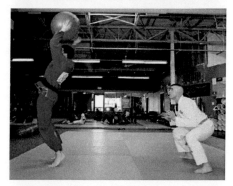

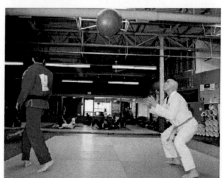

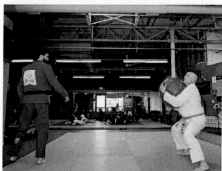

TSW 10 *Lift Jitsu for 4-5 Rounds*

Waterball Throw and Catch

Stand facing away from your partner. Make sure you have plenty of room as well as overhead clearance. Squat with a waterball then explode up, throwing the ball overhead as high and far as possible. Your partner's goal is to catch the ball. It may take a rep or two to guage distance, but you should quickly figure out how far the ball will go. Catching a high flying waterball is part of the challenge. Take it full in the chest and try to control the violent sloshing implement without dropping it or being knocked over.

5 rounds of:

Throw and Catch x 5 throws each
Sparring x 3 minutes

WHAT IS A WATERBALL?

A waterball is simply a stability ball full of water. Start with a ball full of air, then use the nozzle that comes with a package of waterballoons to add as much water as you'd like. We use 25, 40, 60, and 80 lb waterballs. We made a 150 lb. ball once, and it was nearly impossible to use. I fully expect some of you to take that as a challenge. Honestly, I'd be disappointed if you didn't!

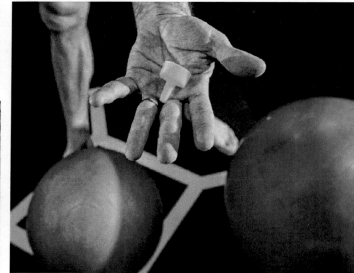

Task Specific Workout 11 - Metabolic Conditioning

TSW 11 *Alternate for as Many Rounds as Possible in 15 Minutes*

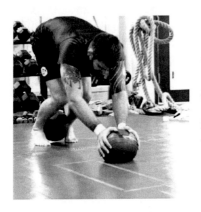 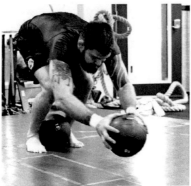 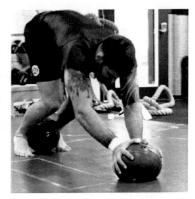

As Many Rounds as Possible in 15 Minutes of:

Medicine Ball Crawl x 10 yds
Waterball Shouldering x 10

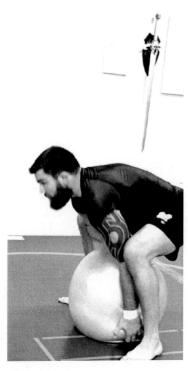 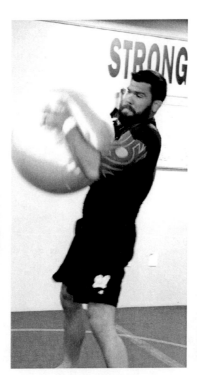 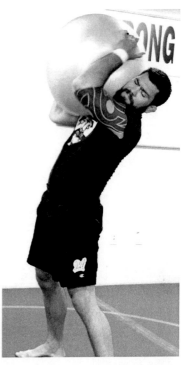

<u>TSW 12</u> *5 rounds of Tire Flip and Car Pull*

5 Rounds of:

Tire Flips x 5-10 (depending on size of tire)
Truck Pull x 30 meters (can push if you don't have a harness)

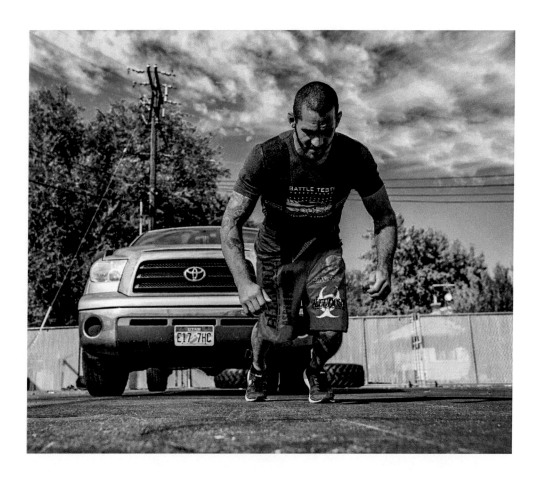

Task Specific Workout 12 - Load Carriage

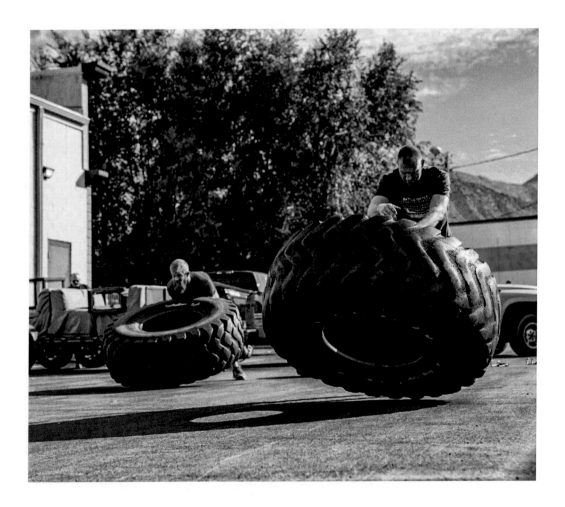

<u>TSW 13</u> *5 Rounds Hand Wrestling, King Crab and Partner Rotation*

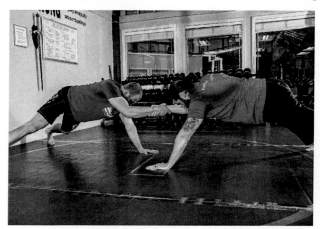 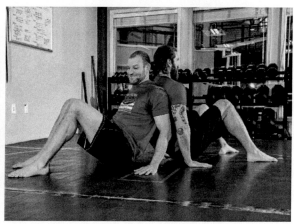

<u>Prone Hand Wrestling</u>

Start in a push-up position facing your partner. Partners grasp right wrists and at the command of go, both partners attempt to pull each other off balance. When one partner hits a knee (or chest, or face), switch hands and repeat. That is one round. Now move on to King Crab.

Alternately, in a group of people, you can run the drill shark tank style, with one athlete going against every other athlete before switching, or include it as the final exercise in a circuit.

<u>King Crab</u>

King Crab is similar to shoulder wrestling where two partners try to force each other out of bounds while in a crab walk position. You can tape lines on the floor, set up cones, or use the pre-marked rings on a wrestling mat. Once you decide the boundaries, both partners begin in the middle of the competition area in a crab walk position with their backs against each other. On the command of go, both partners use their legs to drive backward, trying to force their partner over the boundary line. One round is one minute. Regardless of how many times you or your partner gets pushed out of the boundaries, keep going for the entire minute.

Alternately, in a group of people, you can run the drill shark tank style, with one athlete going against every other athlete before switching, or include it as the final exercise in a circuit.

Task Specific Workout 13 - Partner Exercises

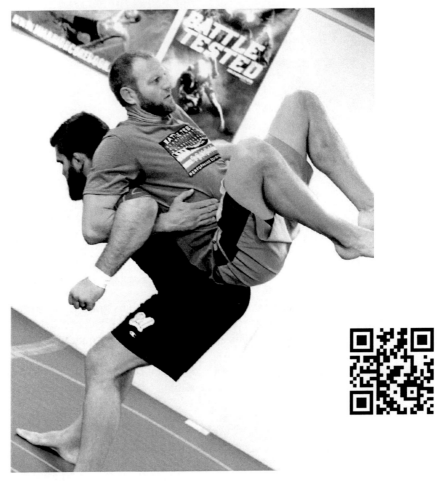

Partner Rotation

Stand back to back and interlock arms with your partner. One partner leans forward while the other pulls his knees up off the floor. Slowly and in control, the bottom partner rotates to the right and left. Rotate slowly back and forth for one minute. Switch places and repeat. This is challenging regardless of which position you are in. One minute in each position equals one round. Rest 1 minute and go back to Prone Hand Wrestling.

<u>TSW 14</u> *Perform for 5 minutes each*

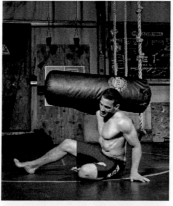

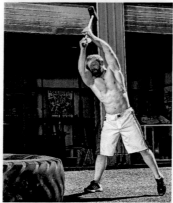

5 minutes of Heavy Bag Turkish Get-ups
Rest 1 minute
5 minutes of Sledge Hammer Swings
Rest 1 minute
5 minutes of Ground and Pound

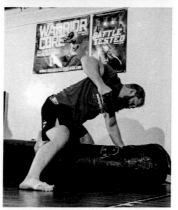

Task Specific Workout 15 - Load Carriage

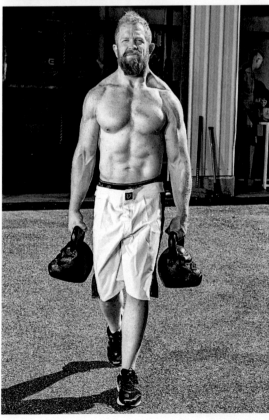

TSW 15 *Perform 8 sets of 8 each*

Squat/Carry/Swing

Place two markers 50 yds. apart. Starting at the first marker, perform 8 repetitions of Kettlebell Goblet Squatts (using 1 kettlebell). Pick up a second kettlebell and perform a 50 yd. Farmer Carry to the second marker. After 50 yds., set one of the kettlebells down and perform 8 Kettlebell Swings with the other kettlebell. After the Kettlebell Swings, pick up the second kettlebell and carry both kettlebells back to the starting point. Continue carrying the kettlebells back and forth until you have have performed 8 sets each of Kettlebell Goblet Squats and Kettlebell Swings.

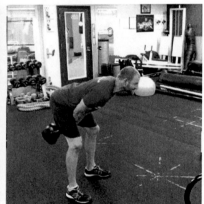

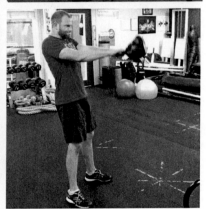

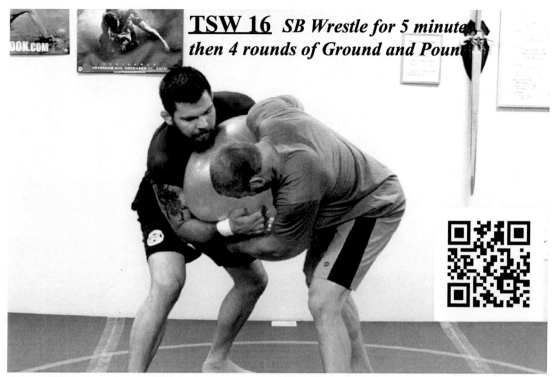

TSW 16 *SB Wrestle for 5 minutes, then 4 rounds of Ground and Pound*

Stability Ball Wrestling

This drill is both fun and exhausting. Make sure you have plenty of room and are a good distance away from any hard objects. It is not unusual for one or both partners to hit the ground during this drill. The rules are simple. Both partners grasp the ball, then on the command of go, do anything they can (excluding biting, foot stomps and shin kicks) to take the ball away from each other.

MMA and TSAC:

This is a 3-5 minute drill. Once someone wins, allow 10-20 seconds of rest before beginning again. Set a timer and continue battling it out for 3-5 minutes. When performing in a group, one person can alternate wrestling everyone else for 3-5 minutes, then a new person is in the middle. 5 minutes of this drill WILL WRECK YOU!

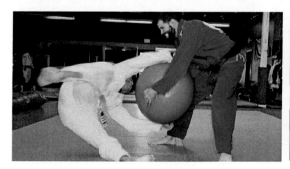
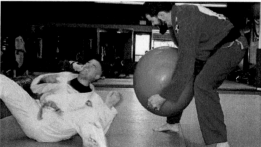

Task Specific Workout 16 - Partner Exercises

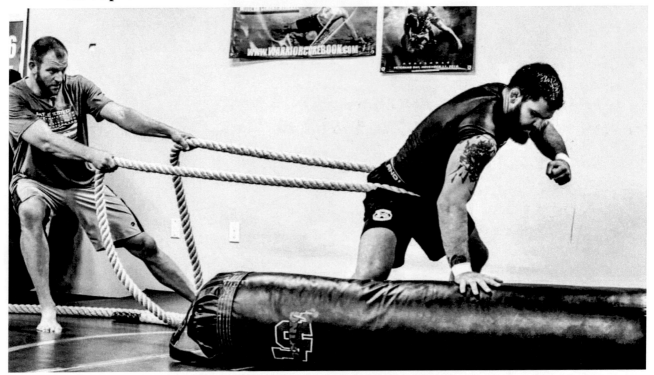

Partner Resisted Ground and Pound

Anyone can strike a bag on the ground. In real life, that person you are trying to hit is going to be fighting back, moving around, and trying for all they are worth to escape. This progression of the Ground and Pound drill I learned from Martial Arts Hall of Famer and CrossFit Striking founder, George Ryan. He taught it with a 2-inch superband around the waist, but with a big strong man like Robert Drysdale, a band is not enough. A battle rope gives you more control over your partner and allows you to pull even harder. Whether you use a band or a rope, this is a fantastic drill and will test your determination like few other drills.

Partner 1 starts with the rope around his waist a short distance from the heavy bag. On the signal go, sprint all out against Partner 2's resistance reaching the bag at any cost. It should be a struggle to get to the bag, but doable. Once Partner 1 reaches the bag, it is business as usual, as he fights to stay in control of the bag and attempts to attack from any angle possible, as Partner 2 tries to pull him off of it. I've literally seen athletes drag the bag with them continuing to throw strikes while their partner pulls them across the mat.

MMA and TSAC:

Again, do this drill in 30 second bouts with 90 seconds rest to start. If you are not tired after 30 seconds, strike harder, transition more and encourage your partner to pull harder! As the drill gets easier, increase time to 45, then 60 seconds. Do 3-4 rounds. Decreasing the rest interval will also make it harder.

TSW 17 *Stadiums - Sprint Up and Bear Crawl Down for 15-20 minutes*

Stadium Up-Downs

Start at one end of the stadium and sprint up the stairs. Jog over to the next set of stairs and bear crawl down. At the bottom, jog over to the next set of stairs and sprint back up. Repeat up and down through all the sets of stairs at the stadium. After the last set, jog back to the start. Repeat for 15-20 minutes. To make this harder, feel free to wear a weight vest. The bear crawls are VERY shoulder intensive, so if you start to fear for your face, jog down, sprint between and bear crawl up.

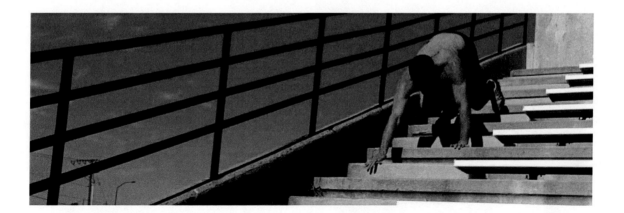

Task Specific Workout 18 - Load Carriage

TSW 18 *Alternate 100 yd. Drags and Zercher Carries for 4-5 rounds*

Zerch and Drag

Alternate dragging a tire or sled for 100 yds. and performing a Barbell Zercher Carry for 100 yds. Be sure to brace your core, drawing in your ribs, and not allowing more than neutral arch of the lumbar spine during the Zercher Carry. The barbell can be loaded with weight plates, or as in the photo below, chains that swing around challenging balance and core stability. A slosh pipe can also be used instead of a barbell to further challenge lateral stability.

Pull the tire or sled as fast as possible. Based on weight of the implement, this can be an all out sprint, or a steady grinding pull. Focus on stability on the Zercher Carry.

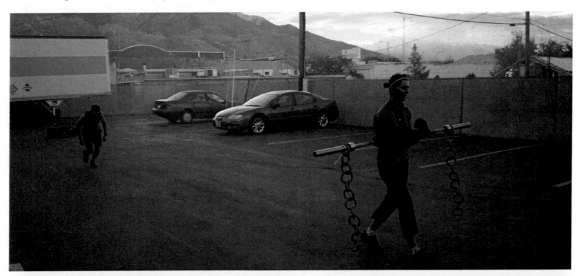

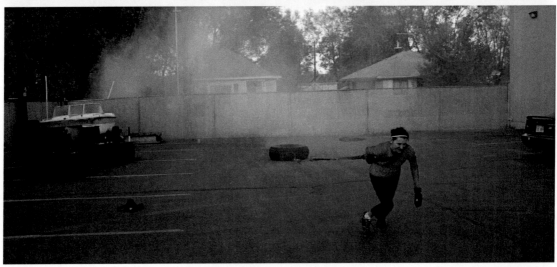

TSW 19 *10 Rounds of 2 Shake-offs and 1 Tire War*

Partner Shake-off

    This exercise begins in nearly the same position as the Partner Get-up. Partner 1 will begin on his hands and knees while Partner 2 climbs on the his back. Partner 2 grabs both underhooks, but does not get the hooks with his feet, rather squeezing his knees against Partner 1's hips.

    Once the position is set, Partner 1 comes off his knees to his hands and feet and proceeds to attempt shaking Partner 2 off of his back. This is challenging for both partners, as Partner 1 moves in a heavily loaded push-up position, and Partner 2 maintains constant tension, squeezing to hold on. Have each partner in each position until the top partner is shaken or the bottom partner collapses, then move immediately to a Tire War.

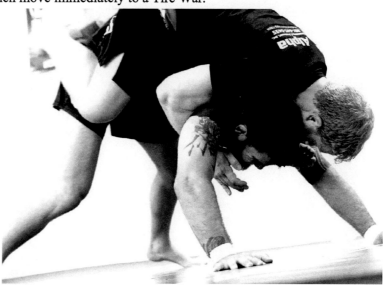

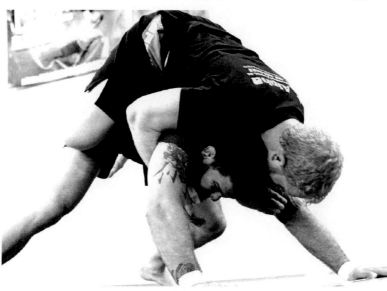

Task Specific Workout 17 - Metabolic Conditioning

Tire War

The tire war is designed to be an explosive all-out effort. This exercise becomes more effective the more competitive it gets, so be aggressive. It trains generating power in the hips and using the whole body to throw the tire at your partner, thus translating well to punching power.

With two athletes on opposing sides of a tire, have one explosively push the tire at the other. The 2nd partner must catch and decelerate the tire before firing it back at the 1st partner. Stand with a staggered stance to improve stability, but feel free to switch stances back and forth. Be sure to brace your core to increase stability and power. A 300-350 lb. tire works great. Because this is a power exercise, keep sets to no more than 30 seconds of 100% effort. Rest 1 minute and go back to the Partner Shake-off. Do 10 rounds.

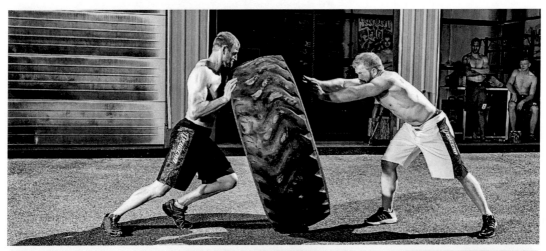

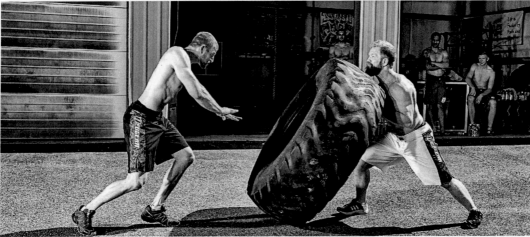

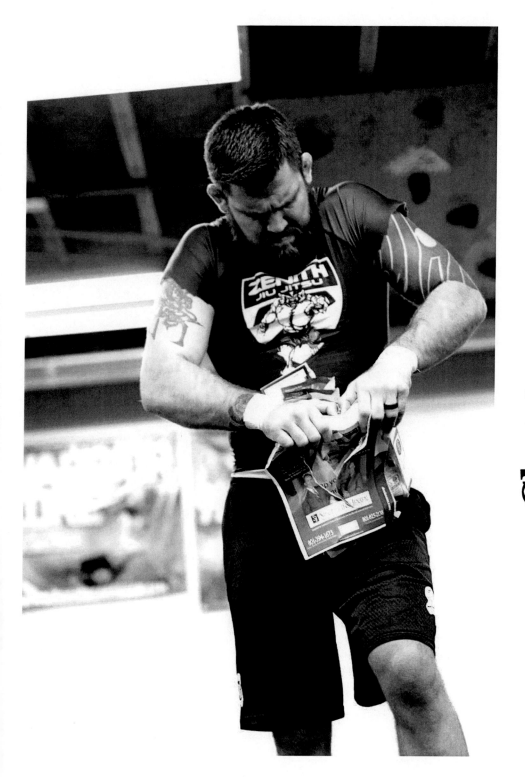

Chapter 12
Grip Training

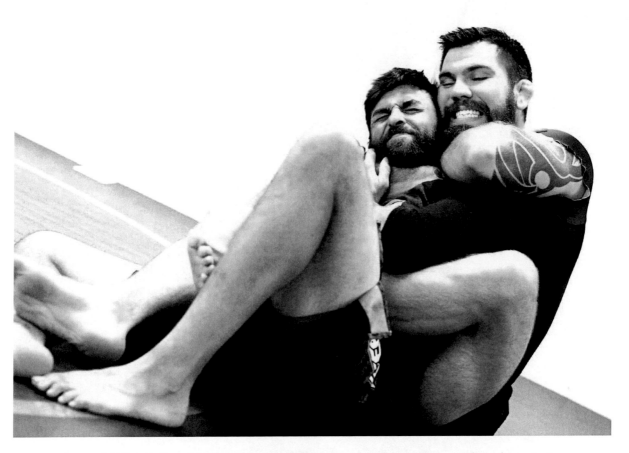

As previously mentioned, both squeeze strength (shown above) and grip strength are important for warriors. In MMA, wrestling and no gi jiu-jitsu, squeeze strength is likely more important. For gi jiu-jitsu, judo, and people who work with firearms, grip strength is more important. Improving your grip strength will also improve your strength in many lifts and things like pull-ups and rope climbs. \

The company IronMind (www.ironmind.com) make the best grip training implements I have ever used and in my mind are the authority on grip training. They have developed a model for grip training called the "Crushed-to-Dust CUBE". The CUBE booklet is available on their website and I encourage you to check it out. The idea is that there are 8 different types of grip training, made up of 2 hand positions (open and closed), 2 prime movers (crush grip and pinch grip), and 2 intensities (1-rep max and endurance). We will classify our movements simply as crush grip or pinch grip.

Each training session, you should pick a grip exercise to do here and there throughout your workout. Be sure to balance crush grip, pinch grip and extensor exercises from workout to workout.

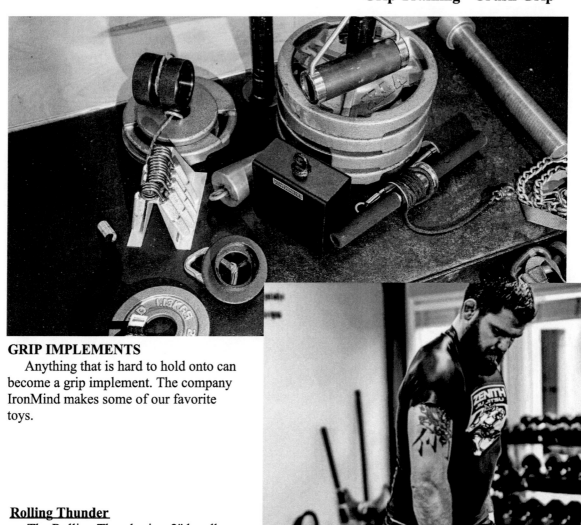

GRIP IMPLEMENTS

Anything that is hard to hold onto can become a grip implement. The company IronMind makes some of our favorite toys.

Rolling Thunder

The Rolling Thunder is a 2" handle that rotates, made by IronMind. Your goal is simply grab the handle and stand up with it with hips and knees locked out for at least 1 second. If successful, add more weight and try again. As you get near your max, rest 2-3 minutes between attempts.

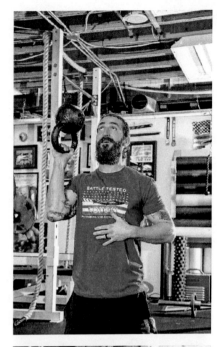

<u>Bottoms-Up KB Press</u> (Also a Vertical Press Exercise)
 Begin by turning a kettlebell upside-down. Grip the handle tightly so that it does not swing down into your wrist. Continuing to hold the kettlebell upside-down, slowly press it overhead.

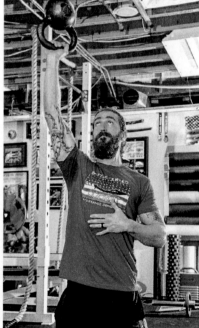

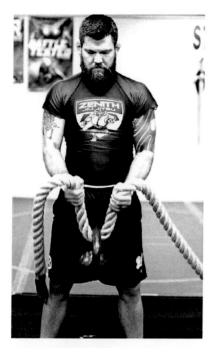

KB Rope Curl

Slide a battle rope through 1-2 kettlebells. Grasp the rope on both sides of the rope with an underhand grip. From here, you will simply be performing a Biceps Curl. Keep your elbows glued to your sides and flex the elbows to bring your hands up to your chin. Slowly control both the concentric (lifting) and eccentric (lowering) portions of the lift.

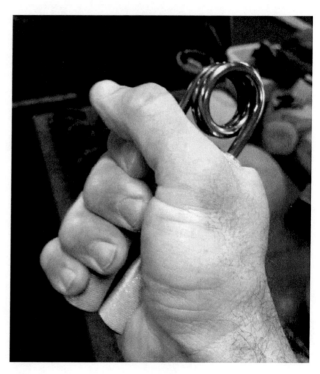

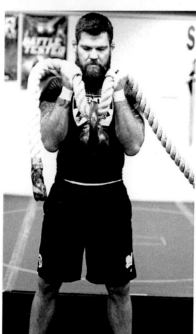

Grippers

Grippers are a common way to improve crush grip strength. Not all grippers are created equal however. Once again, IronMind dominates the competition with their Captains of Crush (COC) grippers. COC grippers range in difficulty from 60-365 lbs! The 60 and 80 lb. grippers are designed for rehab. Iron Mind recommends strong people start with the 100 lb. trainer and working up from there.

Grip Training - Crush Grip

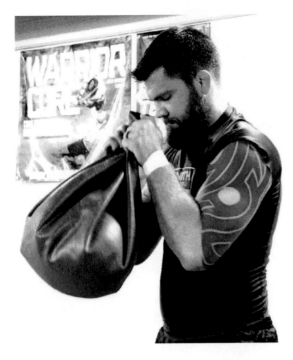

WHAT IS A GRAPPLE GRIPPER?
A grapple gripper is similar to a waterball, it just doesn't have any air in it. Take a flat ball and using the nozzle that comes with a pack of water balloons, fill it with the desired amount of water.

Grapple Gripper Curl
Grasp your grapple gripper with both hands and do Biceps Curls. Keep your elbows glued to your sides and flex the elbows to bring your hands up to your chin. Slowly control both the concentric (lifting) and eccentric (lowering) portions of the lift.

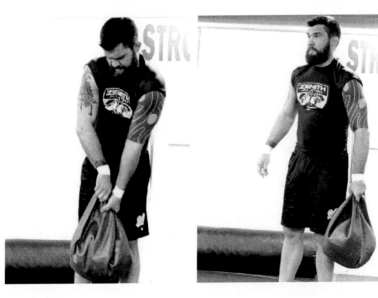

Grapple Gripper Hold
Grasp your grapple gripper with one hand. Hold it as long as possible. Switch hands when necessary.

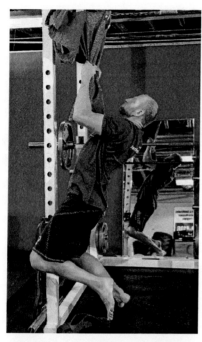

Gi Pull-up (Also a Vertical Pull Exercise)

Using a gi, or a towel draped over a bar makes Pull-ups really hard! Perform just like you would perform a Neutral Grip Pull-up. You can also loop a battle rope over the bar and hold on to that. Your hands will definitely fatigue before your back. For gi competitors in Judo or Jiu-Jitsu, this is a fantastic addition to your training.

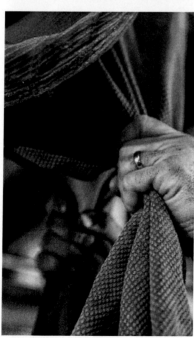

Grip Training - Pinch Grip

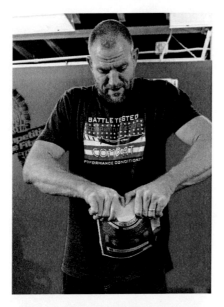

Tearing Phone Books

Tearing phone books is quickly becoming a lost art. Already, phone books are a third of the size they used to be. It is sad really. Phone book tearing is a great pinch grip exercise however, so if you have the opportunity, do it!

First, holding the phone book vertically, place your thumbs on the near-side of the book and your fingers on the outside. Try to make a tight little V with your thumbs as you press the left and right sides of the book towards each other. You want to almost form a crease in the phone book. From here, trying to maintain the V, push your thumbs down and away from each other with a twisting wrist movement. Once you get the pages started tearing, the rest goes pretty easily.

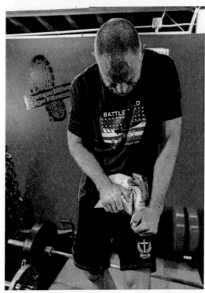

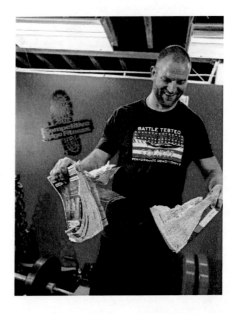

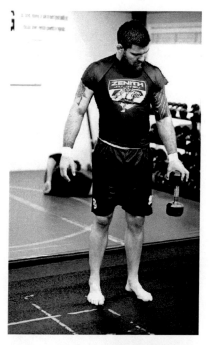

DB End Hold

Grasp a dumbbell by the end and hold for time. With smaller dumbbells, make sure that you are not allowing your finger tips to wrap around to hook the dumbbell. This is a open pinch exercise. If you wrap your fingers around, it is no longer a pinch. The bigger the dumbbell, the harder it is, not only because of the weight increase, but also because it opens the hand more making the pinch more challenging.

Strength: Squat down to lift the dumbbell off the floor. Come to a complete upright position, then set it back down. Don't drop your dumbbells. Not only is it bad for the dumbbells and your toes, it is also lazy.

Endurance: Hold the dumbbell for as long as possible to improve endurance. If you can hold it longer than 30 seconds, consider using a heavier dumbbell. This increases

Circus Tricks: Begin with a dumbbell that you can hold for at least 30 seconds. From a standing position, swing the dumbbell slightly and flick your wrist, releasing the dumbbell to flip it end over end. Catch the dumbbell by the opposite end. Remember, dropping dumbbells is bad for dumbells and toes.

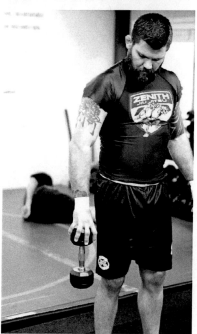

Grip Training - Pinch Grip

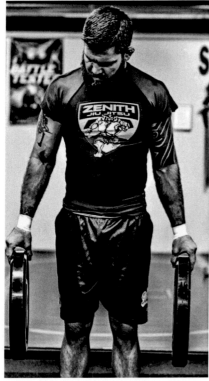

Plate Pinch

Similar to the DB End-Hold, but with bumper plates. Grab a plate in each hand and hold for as long as possible.

Pinch Blocks

You can easily make pinch grip blocks out of a small piece of 2 x 4 or 4 x 4 lumber and an eye screw. I encourage you to make both as the difference in width challenges your grip in a slightly different way. Once you have your blocks, simply use a plate load pin or carabiner and small loop of webbing to attach it to a weight plate.

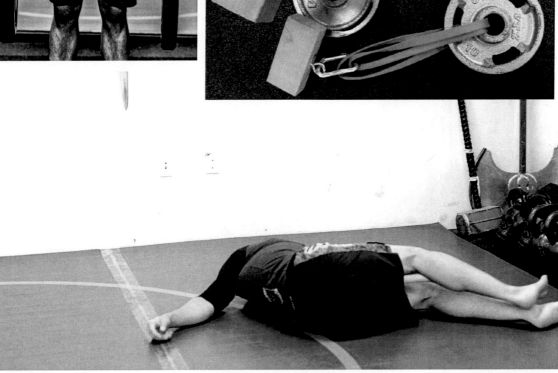

Wrist Roller

One of the most common ways to work the extensors, wrist rollers can be found at most sporting goods stores for a reasonable price. You can also improvise with a barbell on a squat rack with a band and a couple weight plates. The wrist roller works both the flexors (with a crush grip) and the extensors, depending which way you roll it. Both are great, but on extensor days, place special emphasis on bringing the back of your hand towards you forearm. Once you have rolled the weight up to the handle, slowly lower them back down to take advantage of the eccentric contraction as well.

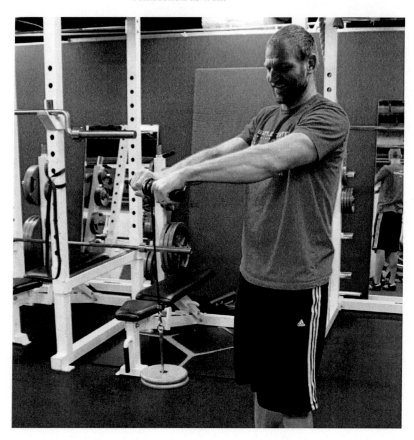

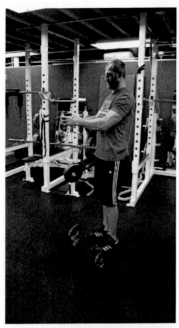

Twist Yo' Wrist

The IronMind Twist Yo' Wrist is essentially a giant yo-yo that you hold upside-down with weight dangling from the string. You then twist your hands at the wrists to roll the string back onto the implement, raising the weight. Reverse the movement, controlling the descent to eccentrically work the muscles. Once the weight is lowered, you continue rotating the implement in the same direction to raise the weight again using the opposite movement. In addition to wrist flextion and extension, this brings ulnar and radial deviation as well as pronation and supination into the mix, making this exercise one of my all-time favorites for wrist and elbow health.

You can also simulate this implement with a small dumbbell, a superband (or loop of webbing) and a few small weight plates.

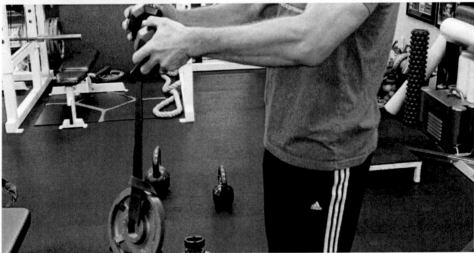

Rice Bucket

Another great way to train hand and wrist strength is with a bucket full of rice. Again, you can use this exercise both for the flexors (crush grip) and for the extensors. We are most concerned with the extensors. With hand open and fingers stretched wide, bury your hand in the bucket of rice. Once your hand is completely buried, squeeze your fingers together, closing your hand into a fist. This works the flexors. Now reverse the movement, opening your fist under the rice and spreading your fingers wide. This trains the extensors. You can also strengthen pronation and supination by rotating your wrist as you squeeze and open your fist.

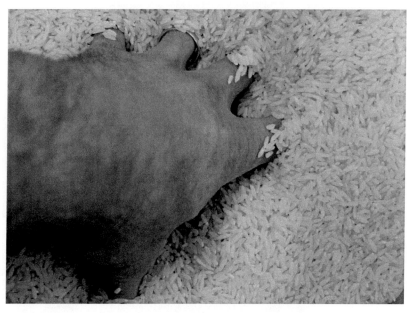

Grip Training - Wrist Extensors

EZ-Curl Bar Wrist Extensions

Another simple exercise to train the wrist extensors is to kneel in front of a bench with your forearms on the bench and your hands hanging palms down off the opposite side. With a curl bar in your hands, slowly lower them into a flexed wrist position. Now reverse the movement, extending the wrists as far as possible to lift the bar up again.

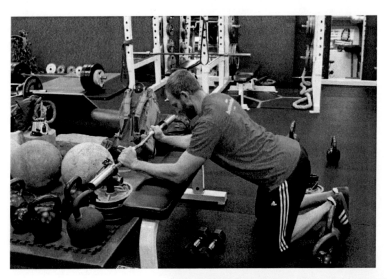

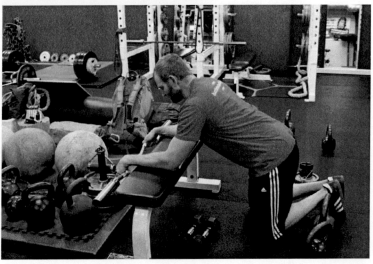

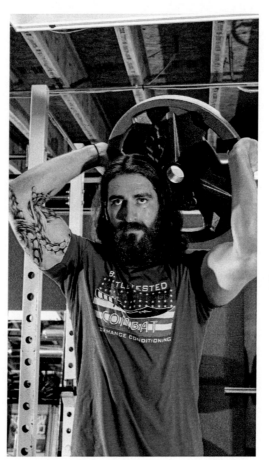

Chapter 13
Finishers

Chapter 12 - Finishers

The finisher is meant to create intense muscular fatigue prior to completing the task, but having to complete the task anyway. My goal is for you to want to quit before you are done, but to stick through it anyway. This is typically done with light to moderate weight for really high repetitions or for a certain amount of time. We do not use exercises during this portion of the workout that are technically difficult. The last thing we want to do is injure ourselves, so we stick with safe exercises that are not technically complex.

There are of course some finishers that are full body, but in general, we will alternate between upper and lower body finishers from workout to workout.

4-Minute Squat

Perform Bodyweight Squats as fast as possible for 20 seconds. Pause AT THE BOTTOM for 10 seconds, then repeat. Perform 8 rounds total or 4 continuous minutes.

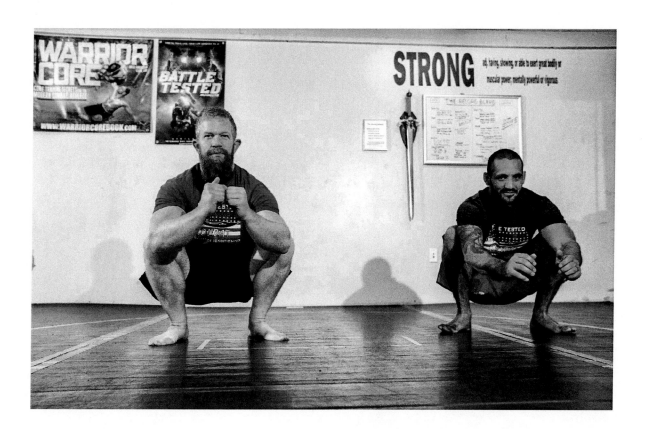

Upper Body Finishers

Plate Floor Press

This finisher is just like the DB Floor Press on page 180, but using a 45 lb. weight plate rather than dumbbells. Your goal is 120 repetitions. You are not allowed to set the plate down, or rest with your elbows on the floor. You can only pause with arms fully extended. The first 60 repetitions are usually fairly easy. After that, it becomes a bit of a mind game. It may get to the point where you can only do 3-4 reps between pauses. No problem. Keep going until you reach 120. Once you can do this, progress to 2 sets of 120, then 3 sets of 120, and finally 3 sets of 150 repetitions.

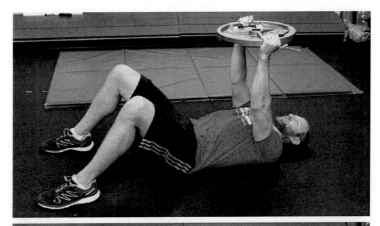

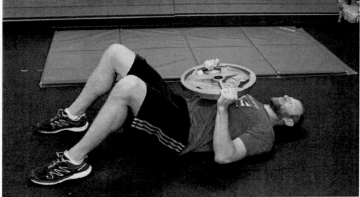

Lower Body Finishers

Kettlebell Swing Breathing Ladder

Perform 1 Kettlebell Swing, rest for 1 breath. Do 2 Kettlebell Swings, rest for 2 breaths. 3 repetitions, then 3 breaths, etc., etc. Work up to 10 repetitions and back down. As you progress, work to 12 repetitions and down and add weight.

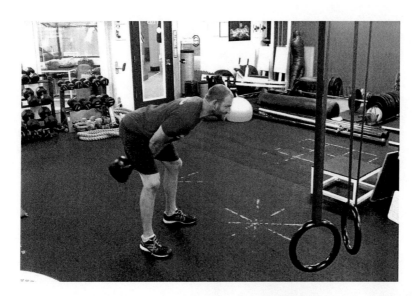

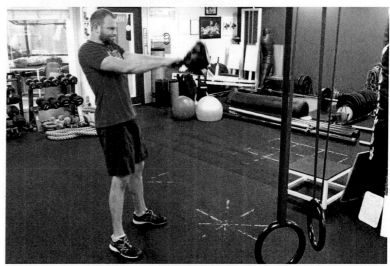

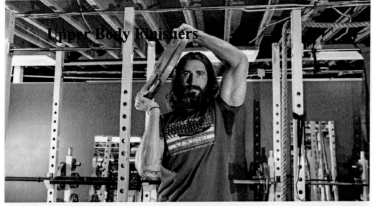

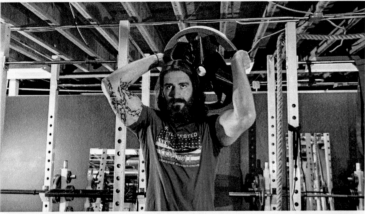

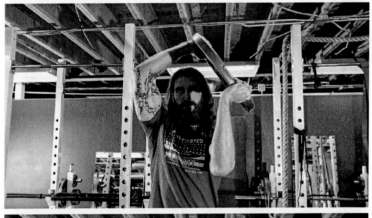

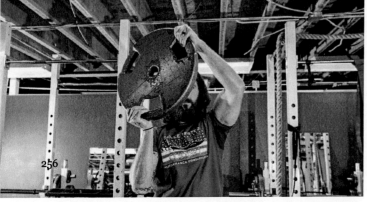

Plate Halo

Plate Halos are very simple. They can be performed standing or sitting. If you have never done halos, start with a 25 lb. weight plate. As your mental durability improves, you can progress to a 35 lb. plate and eventually a 45 lb. plate.

Place your hands directly across the plate from each other. Lift the plate above your head. Bend your elbows and start making tight circles around your head in either direction. Make sure to keep your neck relaxed and move the plate around your head instead of trying to move your head around the weight.

Go for 5 minutes. There is only one rule. DO NOT LOWER THE WEIGHT BELOW YOUR SHOULDERS for the entire 5 minutes! By 2 minutes, you will want to stop. By 3 minutes your shoulders will be screaming for mercy. Don't give in. You are capable, I promise. You can stop making circles at any time and pause with the plate in any position shown in the photos, but do not set the weight down.

This finisher, like most finishers is 100% more tolerable with your battle buddy.

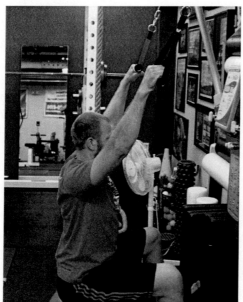

Lat Pull-down

Using a Lat Pull-down machine, set the weight at something you think you can do 20-25 reps on. Then do 50 consecutive repetitions. After 30, you should begin to doubt yourself or the weight is too light. Keep going. Pause if necessary, but do not let go of the handles to release tension of the cable. Your grip, forearms, lats, biceps, and even triceps should be screaming by the time you reach 50.

Rest 2-3 minutes, then repeat for 40 reps. Continue this pattern for 30 reps, 20 reps and 10 reps. On the final set of 10 reps, once you have completed 10, pause at the bottom of the movement for as long as possible. Your goal is to make it AT LEAST a full minute after your 10 repetitons.

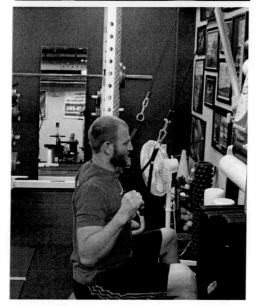

Upper Body Finishers

Alternating 1-arm Superband Row

Using a 1" superband attached to a squat rack, squeeze your shoulder blades together and pull the band to your upper abdomen. Return to the starting position, switch hands and repeat. Continue switching hands every repetition for 5 straight minutes. Be sure to stand far enough back that there is tension on the band when your arm is outstretched in front of you.

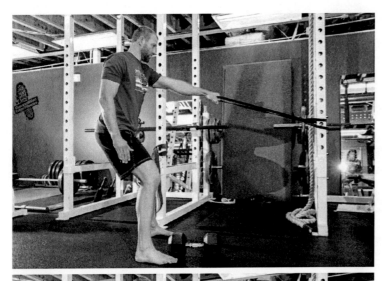

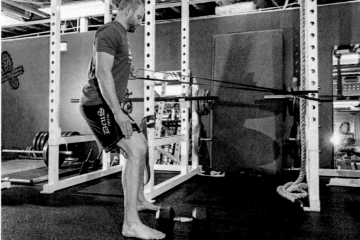

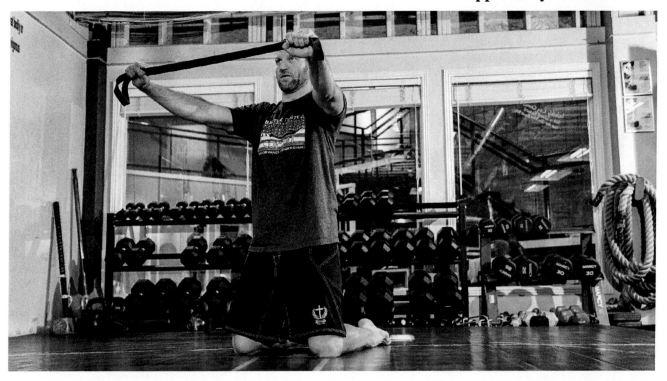

Superband Row/Pullapart

Grab a band for pull-aparts and get a superband set-up for rows. Your goal is 300 repetitions. You may switch exercises anytime that you want to, but try to keep going until you reach a cummulative total of 300 reps.

Upper Body Finishers

Stair Push-up Ladder

Do as many Push-ups as possible in 1 minutes with your hands on the floor. Rest 1 minute. Place your hands on the 1st stair and do as many Push-ups as possible in 1 minute. Rest 1 minute. Place your hands on the 2nd stair and do as many Push-ups as possible in 1 minute.

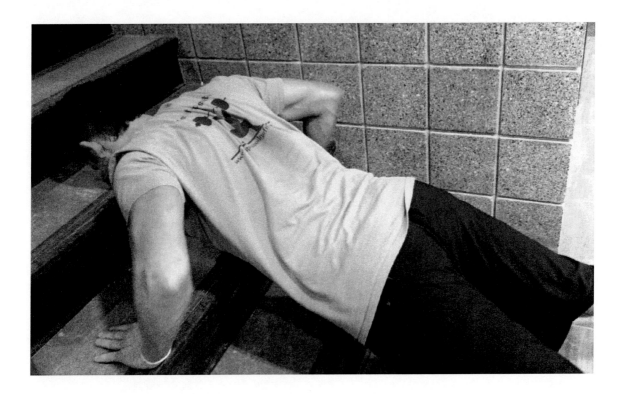

Rope Slam

Grab the ropes with both hands. Stand with your feet hip width apart. Squat slightly then explode upward into triple extension (hips, knees, ankles) while bringing the rope up over your head. Slam the ropes back down as you drop back into a partial squat. Do 300 reps.

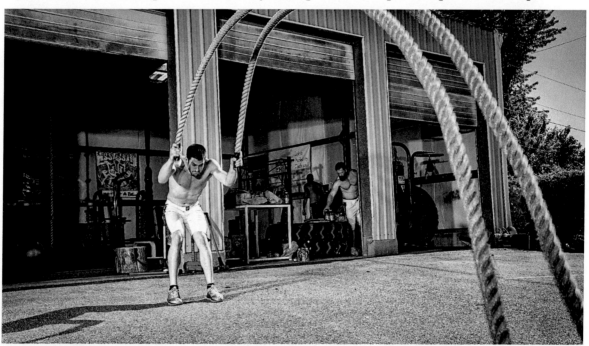

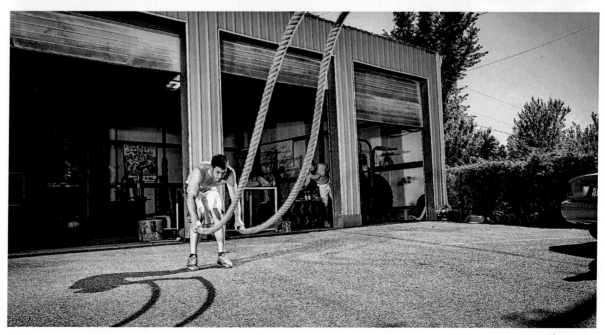

Lower Body Finishers

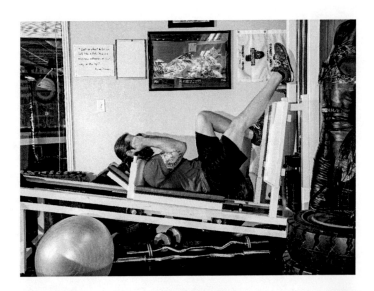

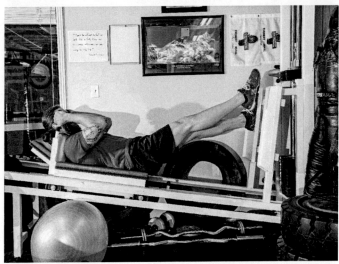

Alternating 1-leg Press

Use a lying leg press machine, perform the press, but using only one leg. To avoid excess stress on the knee, keep your foot up high and drive through your heel, just like on the step-up. Stay stable, not allowing your knee to travel laterally at all.

When you return to the bottom of the movement, switch legs and repeat. Continue alternating legs at the bottom of each repetition for 5 minutes. You can and will slow down, but do not stop.

To progress with this finisher, simply add weight or time. We encourage endurance athletes such as runners, climbers, and mountaineers to work up to 12 minutes.

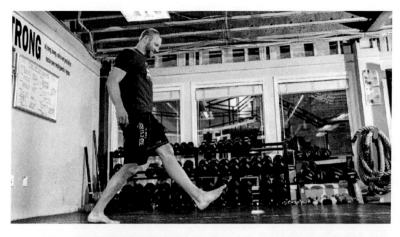

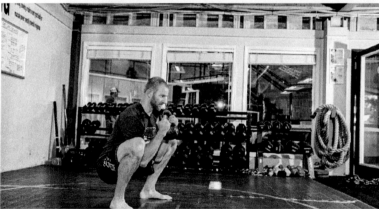

Leg Crank

The Leg Crank is a brutal bodyweight leg circuit that can be done anywhere. If you haven't done them before, start with 1 round. For 1 round, a good time is 90 seconds. Next time you do them, try 2 rounds. The Battle Tested challenge is 4 rounds for time.

Your thighs must hit parallel on all squats and squat jumps. Knees should gently kiss the ground on all lunges and split squat jumps for the time to count. Our current 4-round record is held by retired MMA fighter, Jordan Chandler at 7 minutes and 41 seconds.

If you beat the record (meeting the above criteria) and send us a complete video of the full attempt, we will send you a congratulatory gift. Here we go:

1 Round of Leg Cranks
Bodyweight Squat x 24
Alternating Lunge x 24 (12es)
Split Squat Jump x 24 (12es)
Squat Jump x 24

Lower Body Finishers

Hip Drop 300

The Hip Drop finisher is very similar to the Hip Thrust on page 162. Instead of a bench, put your head and shoulders on a stability ball instead of a bench. The only other difference is that for the Hip Thrust you start on the floor and the Hip Drop you start with your hips in the air. Start with no weight, but as you progress you can begin using a dumbbell. Do as many as you can without resting. If you pause for more than a couple seconds, that is considered a rest.

Every time that you rest, stop, grab 2 heavy dumbbells and climb the nearest stair case. After your DB Stair Climb, start again on the Hip Drop at whatever number you left off. Your goal is to get to 300 repetitions in as few sets as possible.

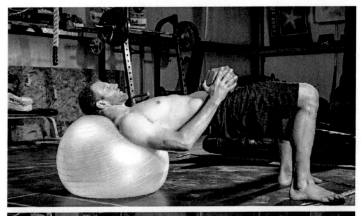

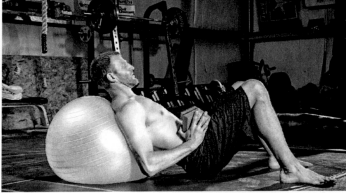

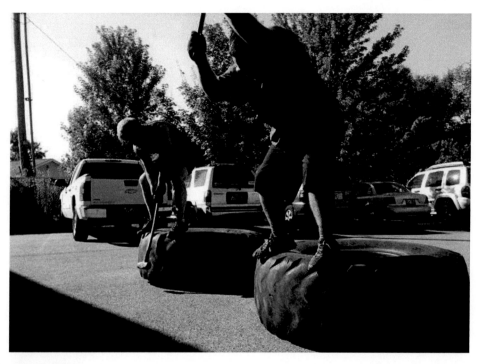

Sledge Hammer Race

The Sledge Hammer Race is one of the most dreaded finishers at our gym. It is more fun with 2 athletes side by side on similar tires with similar hammers, but they can also take turns with one tire. A 300-350 lb. tire and 10-16 lb. sledge works well. Set a timer for 3 minutes. Athletes stand on the edge of the tire and begin swinging the sledge at the tire beneath their feet as hard as they can attempting to move the tire. This is definitely an exercise that involves some technique. It requires a slight hop to unweight the tire as the hammer hits it. Each athlete will figure it out as they go.

The object of the race is to move the tire the furthest in 3 minutes going all out. Within a minute, your entire body will be begging you to stop. Don't.

PART IV
1-Year Battle Tested Program

The program is designed for three days a week, primarily because we expect you to also be doing martial arts or combatives training AT LEAST two or three days a week. Remember the Survival Readiness Triangle? Don't neglect hand-to-hand combat.

If for whatever reason you are not spending time fighting, you may lift four days a week, but follow the same workout order. The workouts are arranged so that they don't interfere with each other if performed more frequently and will even still work great if performed less frequently than the recommended three days a week. This program will follow a progression from stabilization training, to conjugate training, to complex training.

Month 1	**Stabilization**
Months 2, 3, 4	**Conjugate**
Months 5, 6	**Complex**
Month 7	**Stabilization**
Months 8, 9, 10	**Conjugate**
Months 11, 12	**Complex**

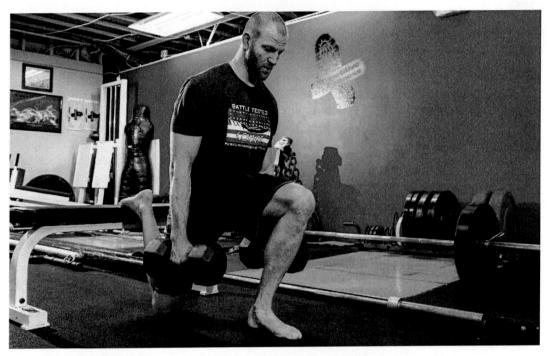

Stability Training Begins Here

The first part of our training year focuses on joint stability and movement mechanics. Essentially, you are going to spend a month bulletproofing basic movements before we add speed and intensity. We will focus on isometrically strengthening the difficult portion of the exercise, which will in turn make it easier during the full speed movements.

Exercises are grouped as A, B, C and sometimes D. You will perform all sets of the A exercises before moving on to the B exercises. A1, A2, A3 are performed one after another as a superset. Do one set of each before moving on to the second set. The first number is always the sets. 4 x 8 means 4 sets of 8 repetitions. 20 x 5 means 20 sets of 5 repetitions.

Stabilization #1

	Week 1	Week 2	Week 3	Week 4
Strength/Power				
A1 Barbell Squat (5s pause at bottom)	4 x 5 @	4 x 6 @	5 x 5 @	4 x 8 @
A2 Push-up (5s pause at bottom)	4 x 5	4 x 6	5 x 6	4 x 8
A3 Dead Bug (each side)	4 x 15s	4 x 20s	5 x 15s	4 x 25s
B1 1-leg Romanian Dead-lift (each side)	4 x 8	4 x 6 @	5 x 6 @	4 x 8 @
B2 Inverted Row (5s pause at top)	4 x 8	4 x 8	5 x 8	4 x 10
B3 Pallof Press (each side)	4 x 5 @	4 x 8 @	5 x 5 @	4 x 8 @
Finisher				
C1 1-leg Alternating Leg Press (switch legs every rep at bottom)	5 min @	6 min @	6 min @	8 min @

Recovery/Regeneration

Stabilization #2

	Week 1	Week 2	Week 3	Week 4
Strength/Power				
A1 Bulgarian Split Squat Hold (each side)	4 x 20s	4 x 30s	5 x 30s	4 x 40s
A2 Savickas Press	4 x 8 @	4 x 10 @	5 x 10 @	4 x 12 @
A3 Core Movement	4 x 12	4 x 15	5 x 15	4 x 20
B1 18-inch DB Step-up (each side)	4 x 8 @	4 x 10 @	5 x 8 @	4 x 12 @
B2 Band Plank Pull Hold (each side)	4 x 15s	4 x 20s	5 x 20s	4 x 30s
B3 Isometric Shoulder Abduction	4 x 30s	4 x 35s	5 x 35s	4 x 45s
Finisher				
C1 Pull-apart/Superband Row (switch exercises as needed)	200 reps	250 reps	300 reps	300 reps

Recovery/Regeneration

Stabilization #3

	Week 1	Week 2	Week 3	Week 4
Strength/Power				
A1 Barbell Hip Thrust (2s pause at top)	4 x 8 @	4 x 10 @	5 x 8 @	5 x 6 @
A2 DB Floor Press	4 x 8 @	4 x 10 @	5 x 8 @	5 x 6 @
A3 Farmer Carry	4 x 40yd	4 x 50yd @	5 x 50yd @	5 x 60yd
B1 KB Goblet Squat	4 x 8 @	4 x 10 @	5 x 8 @	5 x 6 @
B2 Bent-over Row	4 x 12 @	4 x 10 @	5 x 8 @	5 x 6 @
B3 Waiter Carry (each side)	4 x 40yd	4 x 50yd	5 x 50yd	5 x 60yd
Finisherd				
C1 Plank/Side Plank/Boat Pose (switch exercises as needed)	6 min	6 min	8 min	8 min

Recovery/Regeneration

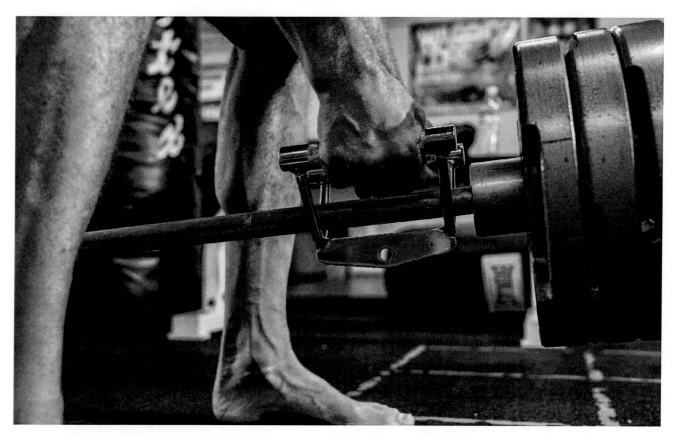

Conjugate Training Begins Here

Conjugate Training essentially alternates heavy, max effort days, fast, dynamic effort days and repetition days. Our task specific portions of the workout and our finishers will take care of the repetition days, so most of of our strength workouts will alternate between max effort upper body, max effort lower body, dynamic effort upper body and dynamic effort lower body. Max effort days are heavy, near max lifts. Dynamic effort days are lifting at 40-60% of 1 repetition max, but focusing on contraction speed. Plyometrics also fit into dynamic effort. Louie Simmons would likely tear this interpretation of Conjugate programming apart - so don't show him.

There are 10 different workouts in this section (40 really, because the task specific and finishers are always changing). Do column 1 of each workout before starting over on column 2.

Battle Tested Program - Conjugate

Conjugate Workout #1 - Max Lower

	#1	#2	#3	#4
Dynamic Warm-up				
Strength/Power		(add weight)	(add weight)	(decrease weight)
A1 Romanian Dead-lift	4 x 8 @	5 x 6 @	6 x 4 @	4 x 6 @
A2 18" DB Step-up	4 x 8es @	5 x 6es @	6 x 4es @	4 x 6es @
A3 Plank Pull	4 x 8es @ 1"	5 x 8es @ 1"	6 x 6es @ 1"	4 x 6es @ 1"
Task Specific				
B1 Task Specific Workout	TSW #1	TSW #13	TSW #6	TSW #18
Finisher				
C1 4-minute Squat	4 min @ No	4 min @ No	4 min @ 20	4 min @ 35
Recovery/Regeneration				

* Grip Training - Pick an extensor training exercise. Do 4-5 sets over the duration of the workout.

Conjugate Workout #2 - Dynamic Upper

	#1	#2	#3	#4
Dynamic Warm-up				
Strength/Power			(add weight)	(add weight)
A1 Landmine Punch Press (% 1RM)	8 x 4es @ 50%	6 x 6es @ 50%	8 x 4es @ 60%	10 x 2es @ 65%
A2 Inverted Row	8 x 4	6 x 6	8 x 6	10 x 4
A3 Reverse Superband Chop	8 x 4es @ 1"	6 x 6es @ 1"	8 x 6es @ 1"	10 x 4es @ 1"
Task Specific				
B1 Task Specific Workout	TSW #2	TSW #14	TSW #7	TSW #19
Finisher				(add weight)
C1 Lat Pull-down	50 reps @	50, 40, @	50, 40, 30, 20, 10	50 reps @
Recovery/Regeneration				

* Grip Training - This finisher will smoke your crush grip. Don't worry about any additional grip work today.

Battle Tested Program - Conjugate

Conjugate Workout #3- Dynamic Lower

	#1	#2	#3	#4
Dynamic Warm-up				
Strength/Power				(add weight)
A1 Barbell Hip Thrust	8 x 2 @	10 x 2 @	12 x 2 @	8 x 2 @
A2 Squat (% 1RM)	8 x 2 @ 60%	10 x 2 @ 55%	12 x 2 @ 50%	8 x 2 @ 65%
A3 KB Russian Twist	8 x 8es @	10 x 6es @	12 x 6es @	8 x 8es @
Task Specific				
B1 Task Specific Workout	TSW #3	TSW #15	TSW #8	TSW #1
Finisher			(add weight)	(add weight)
C1 KB Swing Breathing Ladder	1-10-1 @	1-12-1 @	1-12-1 @	1-8-1 @
Recovery/Regeneration				

* Grip Training - Pick a pinch grip exercise. Do 4-5 sets over the duration of the workout.

Conjugate Workout #4 - Max Upper

	#1	#2	#3	#4
Dynamic Warm-up				
Strength/Power				
A1 Weighted Pull-up (any variation)	15 x 2 @	20 x 2 @	25 x 2 @	12 x 3 @
A2 1-arm DB Floor Press	15 x 2es @	20 x 2es @	25 x 2es @	12 x 3es @
A3 Side Plank Pull	15 x 3es @ 1"	20 x 3es @ 1"	25 x 3es @ 1"	12 x 5es @ 1"
Task Specific				
B1 Task Specific Workout	TSW #4	TSW #16	TSW #9	TSW #2
Finisher				
C1 Stair Push-up Ladder	AMAP	AMAP	AMAP	AMAP
Recovery/Regeneration				

* Grip Training - Weighted pull-ups will challenge your crush grip. Don't worry about any additional grip work today.

Conjugate Workout #5 - Max Lower

	#1	#2	#3	#4
Dynamic Warm-up				
Strength/Power		(add weight)	(add weight)	
A1 Box Squat (18")	5 x 5 @	5 x 4 @	5 x 3 @	6 x 4 @
A2 KB 1-leg RDL	5 x 5es @	5 x 5es @	5 x 5es @	6 x 5es @
A3 Hanging Windshield Wiper	5 x 3es	5 x 4es	5 x 5es	6 x 5es
Task Specific				
B1 Task Specific Workout	TSW #5	TSW #17	TSW #10	TSW #3
Finisher				
C1 SB Hip Thrust	300 reps @ No	300 reps @ 20	300 reps @ 30	350 reps @ No
Recovery/Regeneration				

* Grip Training - Pick an extensor training exercise. Do 4-5 sets over the duration of the workout.

Conjugate Workout #6 - Dynamic Upper

	#1	#2	#3	#4
Dynamic Warm-up				
Strength/Power		(add weight)	(add weight)	
A1 Medicine Ball Slam	8 x 4 @	8 x 4 @	8 x 4 @	10 x 4 @
A2 Bench Press (% 1RM)	8 x 4 @ 50%	8 x 4 @ 55%	8 x 4 @ 60%	10 x 4 @ 45%
A3 Paddleboat	8 x 4es @	8 x 4es @	8 x 4es @	10 x 4es @
Task Specific				
B1 Task Specific Workout	TSW #6	TSW #18	TSW #11	TSW #4
Finisher				
C1 1-arm Alternating Superband Row	5 min @ 1"	5 min @ 1"	6 min @ 1"	8 min @ 1"
Recovery/Regeneration				

* Grip Training - Pick a pinch grip exercise. Do 4-5 sets over the duration of the workout.

Conjugate Workout #7 - Dynamic Lower

	#1	#2	#3	#4
Dynamic Warm-up				
Strength/Power		(add weight)	(add weight)	
A1 Squat Stance Speed Dead-lift (%1RM)	8 x 4 @	8 x 4 @	8 x 4 @	10 x 4 @
A2 Pistol	8 x 4es	8 x 4es @	8 x 4es @	10 x 4es @
A3 Heavy Bag Kick	8 x 4es	8 x 4es	8 x 4es	10 x 4es
Task Specific				
B1 Task Specific Workout	TSW #7	TSW #19	TSW #12	TSW #5
Finisher				
C1 Leg Crank	1 Round	2 Rounds	2 Rounds	3 Rounds
Recovery/Regeneration				

* Grip Training - Pick a crush grip exercise. Do 4-5 sets over the duration of the workout.

Conjugate Workout #8 - Max Upper

	#1	#2	#3	#4
Dynamic Warm-up				
Strength/Power		(add weight)	(add weight)	
A1 DB Floor Press	8 x 4 @	8 x 4 @	8 x 4 @	10 x 4 @
A2 1-arm DB Row	8 x 4es @	8 x 4es @	8 x 4es @	10 x 4es @
A3 Paddleboat	8 x 4es @	8 x 4es @	8 x 4es @	10 x 4es @
Task Specific				
B1 Task Specific Workout	TSW #8	TSW #1	TSW #13	TSW #6
Finisher				
C1 Plate Halo	5 min @ 25	5 min @ 25	5 min @ 35	6 min @ 35
Recovery/Regeneration				

* Grip Training - Pick an extensor training exercise. Do 4-5 sets over the duration of the workout.

Conjugate Workout #9 - Max Lower

	#1	#2	#3	#4
Dynamic Warm-up				
Strength/Power				
A1 Tire Flip	4 x 5	4 x 6	4 x 7	3 x 8
A2 Sledge Hammer Swing	4 x 12es	4 x 12es	4 x 12es	3 x 12es
B1 Truck Pull	2 x As Far As Possible	2 x AFAP	3 x AFAP	4 x AFAP
Task Specific				
B1 Task Specific Workout	TSW #9	TSW #2	TSW #14	TSW #7
Finisher				
C1 Alternating 1-leg Press	5 min @	6 min @	6 min @	8 min @
Recovery/Regeneration				

* Grip Training - Pick a pinch grip exercise. Do 4-5 sets over the duration of the workout.

Conjugate Workout #10 - Dynamic Upper

	#1	#2	#3	#4
Dynamic Warm-up				
Strength/Power				
A1 Box Cross Push-up	4 x 8	4 x 10	4 x 12	5 x 8
A2 Rope Pull	4 x 20yds @	4 x 20yds @	4 x 25yds @	5 x 15yds @
A3 Landmine Rotation	4 x 8 @	4 x 10 @	4 x 12 @	5 x 8 @
Task Specific				
B1 Task Specific Workout	TSW #10	TSW #3	TSW #15	TSW #8
Finisher				
C1 Plate Floor Press	1 x 120 @ 45	2 x 120 @ 45	3 x 120 @ 45	3 x 150 @ 45
Recovery/Regeneration				

* Grip Training - Pick a crush grip exercise. Do 4-5 sets over the duration of the workout.

Build-a-Beast Template

Conjugate Workout #11 - Dynamic Lower

	#1	#2	#3	#4
Dynamic Warm-up				
Strength/Power		(add height)		(add height)
A1 Box Jump	5 x 2 @	4 x 2 @	6 x 2 @	4 x 2 @
A2 Split Squat Jump	5 x 8	4 x 10	6 x 6	4 x 8
A3 Pallof Press	5 x 5es	4 x 8es	6 x 4es	4 x 8es
Task Specific				
B1 Task Specific Workout	TSW #11	TSW #4	TSW #16	TSW #9
Finisher				
C1 Sledge Hammer Race	3 min	3 min	3 min	3 min
Recovery/Regeneration				

* Grip Training - Pick an extensor training exercise. Do 4-5 sets over the duration of the workout.

Conjugate Workout #12 - Max Upper

	#1	#2	#3	#4
Dynamic Warm-up				
Strength/Power		(add weight)	(add weight)	
A1 Savickas Press	5 x 5 @	6 x 4 @	8 x 3 @	10 x 2 @
A2 KB Rope Row	5 x 5 @	6 x 5 @	8 x 5@	10 x 5 @
A3 G Twist	5 x 5es@	6 x 4es @	8 x 3es @	10 x 3es @
Task Specific				
B1 Task Specific Workout	TSW #12	TSW #5	TSW #17	TSW #10
Finisher				
C1 Rope Slam	300 reps	300 reps	320 reps	350 reps
Recovery/Regeneration				

* Grip Training - Pick a pinch grip exercise. Do 4-5 sets over the duration of the workout.

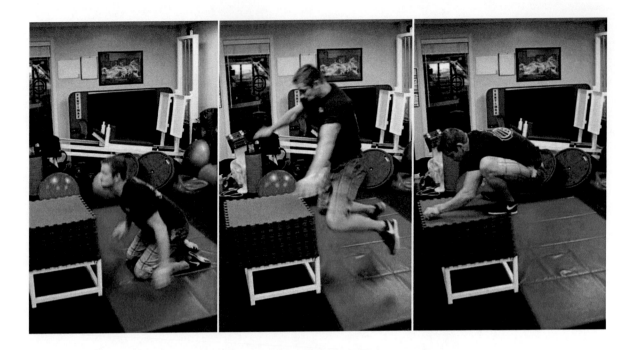

Complex Training Begins Here

Complex training is similar to Conjugate in that it includes max effort and dynamic effort movements, however they are paired together. By doing this, you are able to activate more muscle fibers with a heavy lift that stay activated when you perform your dynamic movement within 60-90 seconds of the heavy lift. We will also be doing some minor agility work in this section, using the Box 5 footwork pattern on pages 158 and 159.

Complex Workout #1

	#1	#2	#3	#4
Dynamic Warm-up				
Box 5 Drills (page 158-159)	Session 1	Session 4	Session 7	
Strength/Power		(add weight)	(add weight)	
A1 Dead-lift	5 x 5 @	6 x 4 @	8 x 3 @	10 x 2 @
A2 Ninja Jump	5 x 5 @	6 x 5 @	8 x 5@	10 x 5 @
A3 G Twist	5 x 5es@	6 x 4es @	8 x 3es @	10 x 3es @
Task Specific				
B1 Task Specific Workout	TSW #11	TSW #17	TSW #4	TSW #9
Finisher				
C1 4-minute Squat	4 min @ 25	4 min @ 30	4 min @ 20	4 min @ 35
Recovery/Regeneration				

* Grip Training - Dead-lifts will challenge your crush grip. Go double overhand as long as possible (until the weight demands mix grip). Don't worry about additional grip work today.

Complex Workout #2

	#1	#2	#3	#4
Dynamic Warm-up				
Strength/Power				
A1 Archer	5 x 6 @	6 x 6 @	8 x 4 @	10 x 4 @
A2 Medicine Ball Slam	5 x 8 @	6 x 8 @	8 x 6 @	10 x 4 @
A3 WB Lunge Twist	5 x 8 @	6 x 8 @	8 x 6 @	10 x 4 @
Task Specific				
B1 Task Specific Workout	TSW #12	TSW #18	TSW #5	TSW #10
Finisher				
C1 Lat Pull-down	2 x 50 @	3 x 50 @	3 x 50 @	50,40,30,20,10 @
Recovery/Regeneration				

* Grip Training - Pick an extensor training exercise. Do 4-5 sets over the duration of the workout.

Complex Workout #3

	#1	#2	#3	#4
Dynamic Warm-up				
Box 5 Drills (page 158-159)	Session 2	Session 5	Session 8	
Strength/Power		(add weight)	(add weight)	
A1 Rack Pull	8 x 2 @	8 x 2 @	10 x 1 @	6 x 3 @
A2 Box Jump	8 x 2 @	8 x 2 @	10 x 1 @	6 x 3 @
A3 Side Plank Press	8 x 4es@	8 x 4es @	10 x 4es @	6 x 6es @
Task Specific				
B1 Task Specific Workout	TSW #13	TSW #19	TSW #6	TSW #11
Finisher			(add weight)	(add weight)
C1 KB Swing Breathing Ladder	1-12-1 @	1-12-1 @	1-12-1 @	1-12-1 @
Recovery/Regeneration				

* Grip Training - Pick a pinch grip exercise. Do 4-5 sets over the duration of the workout.

Complex Workout #4

	#1	#2	#3	#4
Dynamic Warm-up				
Strength/Power		(add weight)	(add weight)	
A1 Push Press	5 x 5 @	6 x 4 @	8 x 3 @	10 x 2 @
A2 Rope Climber (2 rope lengths)	5 x 2 @	6 x 2 @	8 x 2 @	10 x 2 @
A3 Heavy Bag Kick	5 x 5es@	6 x 4es @	8 x 3es @	10 x 3es @
Task Specific				
B1 Task Specific Workout	TSW #14	TSW #1	TSW #6	TSW #12
Finisher				
C1 Stair Push-up Ladder	AMAP	AMAP	AMAP	AMAP
Recovery/Regeneration				

* Grip Training - Pick a crush grip exercise. Do 4-5 sets over the duration of the workout.

Complex Workout #5

Dynamic Warm-up	#1	#2	#3	#4
Box 5 Drills (page 158-159)	Session 3	Session 6		
Strength/Power		(add weight)	(add weight)	
A1 24" Box Squat	8 x 5 @	8 x 4 @	8 x 3 @	10 x 4 @
A2 Split Squat Jump	8 x 6 @	8 x 6	8 x 6	10 x 4
A3 Reverse Superband Chop	8 x 4es@1"	8 x 6es @ 1"	8 x 6es @ 1"	10 x 4es @ 1"
Task Specific				
B1 Task Specific Workout	TSW #15	TSW #2	TSW #7	TSW #13
Finisher				
C1 SB Hip Thrust	300 reps @ 25	300 reps @ 35	300 reps @ 40	350 reps @ 20
Recovery/Regeneration				

* Grip Training - Pick an extensor training exercise. Do 4-5 sets over the duration of the workout.

Complex Workout #6

Dynamic Warm-up	#1	#2	#3	#4
Strength/Power		(add weight)	(add weight)	
A1 DB Floor Press	5 x 5 @	6 x 4 @	8 x 4 @	10 x 4 @
A2 Box Cross Push-up	5 x 8	6 x 8	8 x 6	10 x 4
A3 Side Plank Pull	5 x 8es@	6 x 8es @	8 x 6es @	10 x 4es @
Task Specific				
B1 Task Specific Workout	TSW #16	TSW #3	TSW #8	TSW #14
Finisher				
C1 1-arm Alternating Superband Row	6 min @ 1"	8 min @ 1"	6 min @ 1"	8 min @ 1"
Recovery/Regeneration				

* Grip Training - Pick a pinch grip exercise. Do 4-5 sets over the duration of the workout.

Congrautlations on Completing the
first 6 months of the Battle Tested Program!

Now, start over on the Stabilization portion of
the workout found on page 268. For the next 6
months you will go through the program again,
raising the weight on EVERYTHING!

Once you have gone through the full year (or if
you want to start getting creative now), you can
move on to building your own workouts with the
Build-a-Beast template on the following pages.

PART V
The Build-a-Beast Template

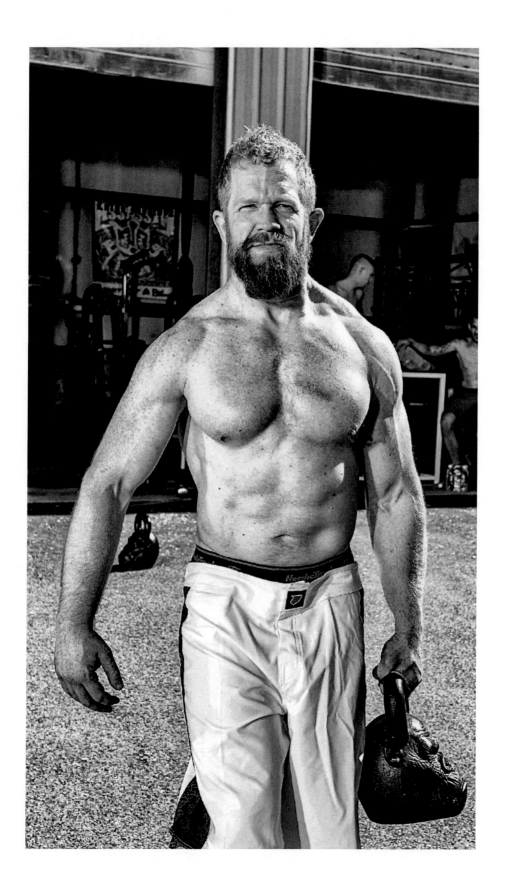

The Build-A-Beast Template

The Build-a-Beast Template

While this book includes a full year of programming, the possible workout combinations can keep you busy for years to come. The following is a template you can use, simply plugging listed exercises and drills in to meet your goals. I encourage you to mix it up, try different combinations, and plan your own workouts. The program is designed for three days a week, primarily because we expect you to also be doing martial arts or combatives training AT LEAST two or three days a week. Remember the Survival Readiness Triangle? Don't neglect hand-to-hand combat. If for whatever reason you are not spending time fighting, you may lift four days a week, but follow the same workout order. The workouts are arranged so that they don't interfere with each other if performed more frequently and will even still work great if performed less frequently than the recommended three days a week.

As with the pre-designed program, the template will follow the same progression from stabilization training, to conjugate training, to complex training.

Month 1	**Stabilization**
Months 2, 3, 4	**Conjugate**
Months 5, 6	**Complex**
Month 7	**Stabilization**
Months 8, 9, 10	**Conjugate**
Months 11, 12	**Complex**

Stabilization #1

Strength/Power	Week 1	Week 2	Week 3	Week 4
A1 Isometric Quad Dominant	4 x 20s	4 x 30s	5 x 30s	4 x 40s
A2 Isometric Horizontal Push	4 x 20s	4 x 30s	5 x 30s	4 x 40s
A3 Isometric Core	4 x 30s	4 x 45s	5 x 45s	4 x 1 min
B1 1-leg Isometric Hip Dominant	4 x 20s	4 x 30s	5 x 30s	4 x 40s
B2 Isometric Horizontal Pull	4 x 15s	4 x 20s	5 x 20s	4 x 30s
B3 Isometric Core	4 x 30s	4 x 45s	5 x 45s	4 x 1 min

Finisher
   C1 Lower Body Finisher

Recovery/Regeneration

Stabilization #2

Strength/Power	Week 1	Week 2	Week 3	Week 4
A1 Isometric Hip Dominant	4 x 20s	4 x 30s	5 x 30s	4 x 40s
A2 Vertical Push	4 x 8	4 x 10	5 x 10	4 x 12
A3 Core Movement	4 x 12	4 x 15	5 x 15	4 x 20
B1 1-leg Quad Dominant	4 x 8	4 x 10	5 x 10	4 x 12
B2 Isometric Vertical Pull	4 x 20s	4 x 30s	5 x 30s	4 x 40s
B3 Shoulder Stability	4 x 12	4 x 12	5 x 12	4 x 15

Finisher
   C1 Upper Body Finisher

Recovery/Regeneration

Stabilization #3

	Week 1	Week 2	Week 3	Week 4
Strength/Power				
A1 Hip Dominant Movement	4 x 8	4 x 10	5 x 8	5 x 6
A2 Horizontal Push Movement	4 x 8	4 x 10	5 x 8	5 x 6
A3 Loaded Carry	4 x 40yd	4 x 50yd	5 x 50yd	5 x 60yd
B1 Quad Dominant Movement	4 x 8	4 x 10	5 x 8	5 x 6
B2 Horizontal Pull Movmenet	4 x 12	4 x 10	5 x 8	5 x 6
B3 Overhead Carry	4 x 40yd	4 x 50yd	5 x 50yd	5 x 60yd

Finisher
    C1 Core Finisher

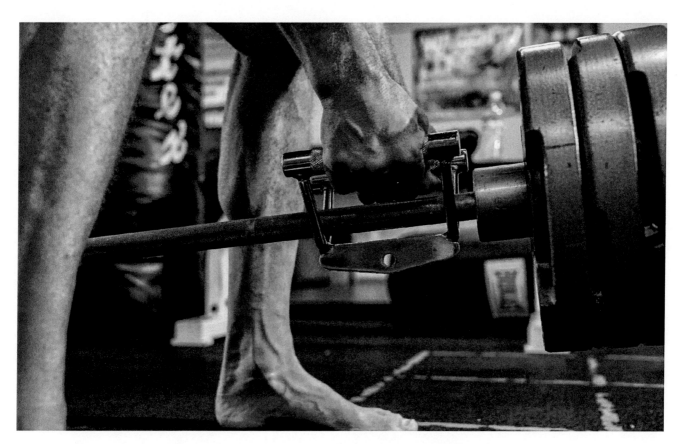

Conjugate Training Begins Here

Build-a-Beast Template

Conjugate - Max Lower #1

Dynamic Warm-up

Strength/Power
   A1 Hip Dominant Movement
   A2 1-leg Quad Dominant
   A3 Core Movement

Task Specific
   B1 MMA or TSAC Specific Drills

Finisher
   C1 Lower Body Finisher

Recovery/Regeneration

Conjugate - Dynamic Upper #1

Dynamic Warm-up

Strength/Power
   A1 Vertical Push (Lift or Throw)
   A2 Horizontal Pull
   A3 Core Movement

Task Specific
   B1 MMA or TSAC Specific Drills

Finisher
   C1 Upper Body Finisher

Recovery/Regeneration

Conjugate - Dynamic Lower #1

Dynamic Warm-up

Strength/Power
   A1 Hip Dominant Movement
   A2 Quad Dominant Movement
   A3 Core Movement

Task Specific
   B1 MMA or TSAC Specific Drills

Finisher
   C1 Lower Body Finisher

Recovery/Regeneration

Conjugate - Max Upper #1

Dynamic Warm-up

Strength/Power
   A1 Vertical Pull
   A2 1-arm Horizontal Push
   A3 Core Movement

Task Specific
   B1 MMA or TSAC Specific Drills

Finisher
   C1 Upper Body Finisher

Recovery/Regeneration

Conjugate - Max Lower #2

Dynamic Warm-up

Strength/Power
    A1 Quad Dominant Movement
    A2 1-leg Hip Dominant
    A3 Core Movement

Task Specific
    B1 MMA or TSAC Specific Drills

Finisher
    C1 Lower Body Finisher

Recovery/Regeneration

Conjugate - Dynamic Upper #2

Dynamic Warm-up

Strength/Power
    A1 Vertical Pull (Lift or Slam)
    A2 Horizontal Push
    A3 Core Movement

Task Specific
    B1 MMA or TSAC Specific Drills

Finisher
    C1 Upper Body Finisher

Recovery/Regeneration

Conjugate - Dynamic Lower #2

Dynamic Warm-up

Strength/Power
   A1 Hip Dominant Movement
   A2 1-leg Quad Dominant
   A3 Core Movement

Task Specific
   B1 MMA or TSAC Specific Drills

Finisher
   C1 Lower Body Finisher

Recovery/Regeneration

Conjugate - Max Upper #2

Dynamic Warm-up

Strength/Power
   A1 Horizontal Push (Lift or Throw)
   A2 1-arm Horizontal Pull
   A3 Core Movement

Task Specific
   B1 MMA or TSAC Specific Drills

Finisher
   C1 Upper Body Finisher

Recovery/Regeneration

Conjugate - Max Lower #3

Dynamic Warm-up

Strength/Power
  A1 Strongman

Task Specific
  B1 MMA or TSAC Specific Drills

Finisher
  C1 Lower Body Finisher

Recovery/Regeneration

Conjugate - Dynamic Upper #3

Dynamic Warm-up

Strength/Power
  A1 Horizontal Push (Lift or Throw)
  A2 Horizontal Pull
  A3 Core Movement

Task Specific
  B1 MMA or TSAC Specific Drills

Finisher
  C1 Upper Body Finisher

Recovery/Regeneration

Conjugate - Dynamic Lower #3

Dynamic Warm-up

Strength/Power
    A1 Quad Dominant Movement (lift or jump)
    A2 1-leg Hip Dominant
    A3 Core Movement

Task Specific
    B1 MMA or TSAC Specific Drills

Finisher
    C1 Lower Body Finisher

Recovery/Regeneration

Conjugate - Max Upper #3

Dynamic Warm-up

Strength/Power
    A1 Vertical Push
    A2 Horizontal Pull
    A3 Core Movement

Task Specific
    B1 MMA or TSAC Specific Drills

Finisher
    C1 Upper Body Finisher

Recovery/Regeneration

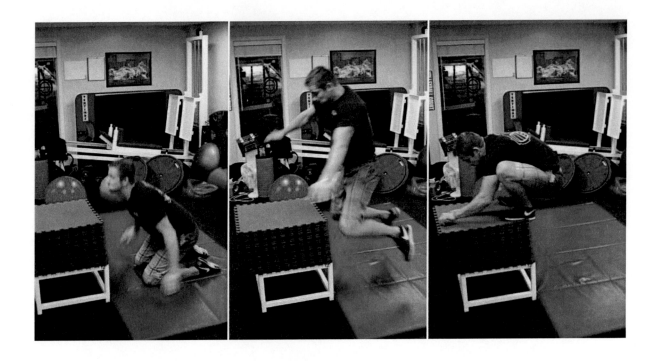

Complex Training Begins Here

Complex #1

Dynamic Warm-up

Box 5 Drills

Strength/Power
  A1 Hip Dominant Heavy
  A2 Hip Dominant Fast
  A3 Core Movement

Task Specific
  B1 MMA or TSAC Specific Drills

Finisher
  C1 Upper Body Finisher

Recovery/Regeneration

Complex #2

Dynamic Warm-up

Strength/Power
  A1 Vertical Pull Heavy
  A2 Vertical Pull Fast
  A3 Core Movement

Task Specific
  B1 MMA or TSAC Specific Drills

Finisher
  C1 Upper Body Finisher

Recovery/Regeneration

Complex #3

Dynamic Warm-up

Box 5 Drills

Strength/Power
    A1 Knee Dominant Heavy
    A2 Knee Dominant Fast
    A3 Core Movement

Task Specific
    B1 MMA or TSAC Specific Drills

Finisher
    C1 Upper Body Finisher

Recovery/Regeneration

Complex #4

Dynamic Warm-up

Strength/Power
    A1 Horizontal Push Heavy
    A2 Horizontal Push Fast
    A3 Core Movement

Task Specific
    B1 MMA or TSAC Specific Drills

Finisher
    C1 Upper Body Finisher

Recovery/Regeneration

Complex #5

Dynamic Warm-up

Box 5 Drills

Strength/Power
  A1 Hip Dominant Heavy
  A2 1-leg Knee Dominant Fast
  A3 Core Movement

Task Specific
  B1 TSAC or MMA Specific Drills

Finisher
  C1 Upper Body Finisher

Recovery/Regeneration

Complex #6

Dynamic Warm-up

Strength/Power
  A1 Horizontal Pull
  A2 Vertical Push Fast
  A3 Core Movement

Task Specific
  B1 MMA or TSAC Specific Drills

Finisher
  C1 Upper Body Finisher

Recovery/Regeneration

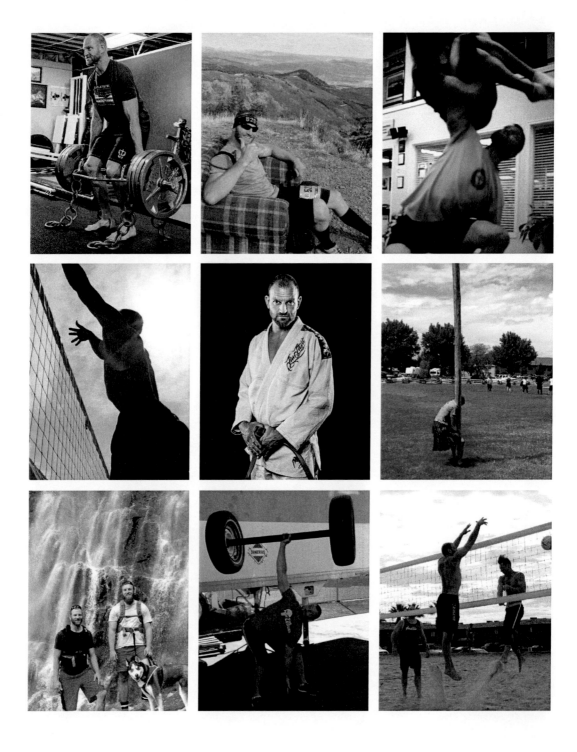

About the Author

ARLO GAGESTEIN

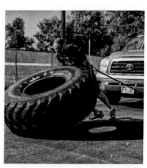

Owner of Competitive Edge Fitness
Fitness Consultant for Ogden City Police
Ground Fighting Instructor for Ogden City Police
Bachelor's Degree in Human Performance
Licensed Sports Massage Therapist
Certified Strength and Conditioning Specialist
Certified MMA Conditioning Coach
Certified Sports Injury Specialist
Certified Core Training Specialist
Brazilian Jiu-Jitsu Purple Belt

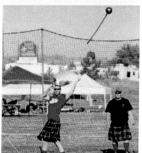

Author of Warrior Core
Published in print and online by:
NSCA Tactical Strength and Conditioning Journal,
MensHealth.com, Jiu-Jitsu Magazine, JJM 360,
Special-Ops Magazine, Fight Camp Conditioning,
Flo Lifestyle, Performance Conditioning Volleyball,
Jiu-JitsuAdvantage.Ninja, and Month 2 Marathon.

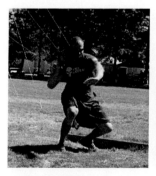
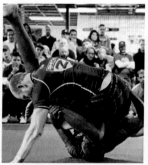
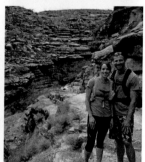
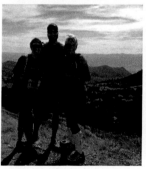
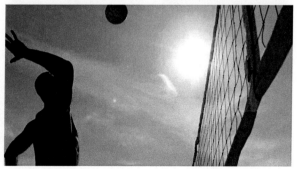